yin yoga

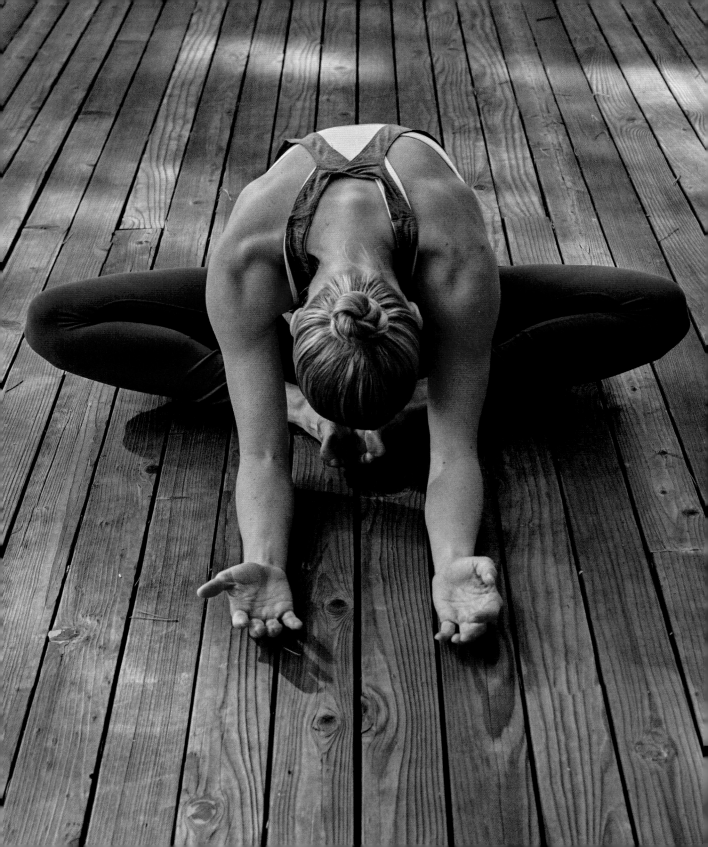

yin yoga

stretch the mindful way

Kassandra
Reinhardt

Contents

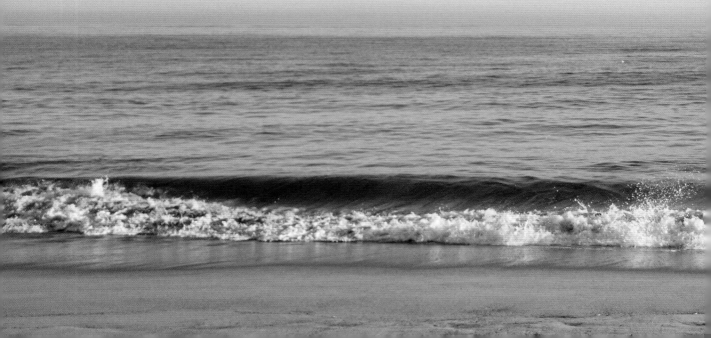

Yin sequences

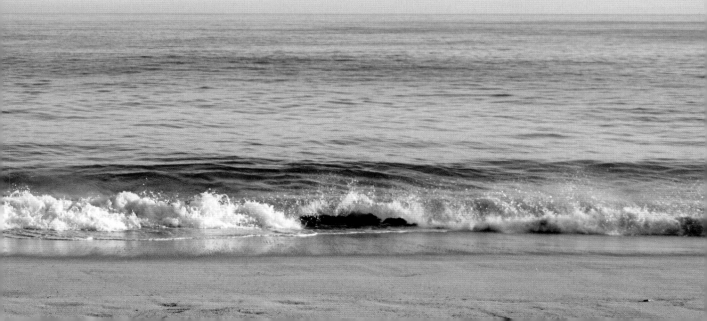

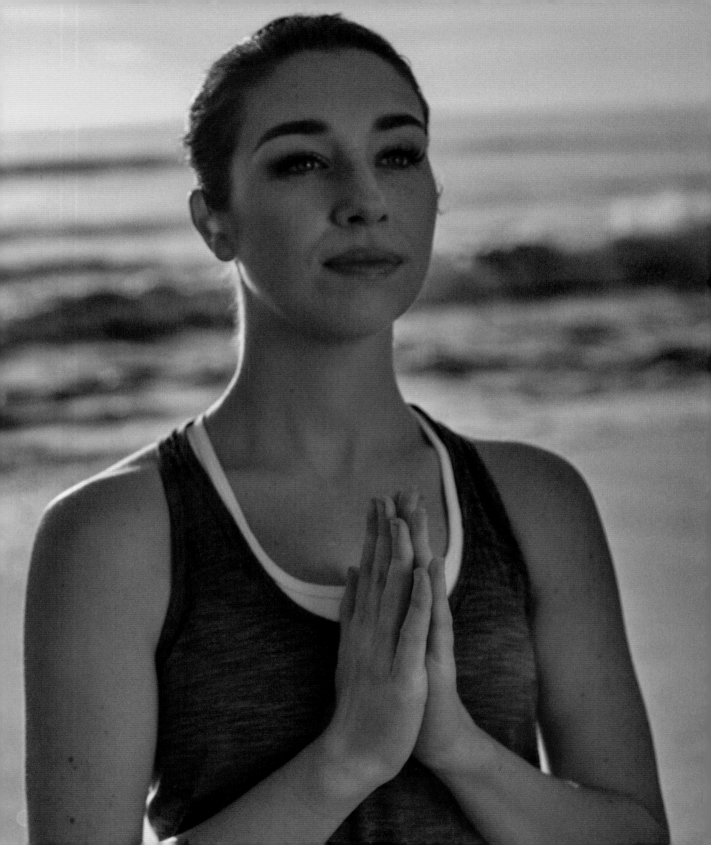

Welcome to yin yoga

Please join me on this journey to learn about this slow-paced style of yoga that can provide a gateway to a way of life filled with more relaxation, greater mindfulness—and less stress. While other yoga forms might push you to strengthen and tone your body, yin yoga invites you to be exactly as you are.

Yin yoga has something to offer to everyone regardless of your reason for picking up this book and getting on your yoga mat. If you're interested in the physical practice of yoga, you'll enjoy the added flexibility and joint health you feel. But if it's the emotional and mental benefits you seek, you'll find techniques to increase your mindfulness and to decrease your stress.

For years, I only practiced stronger styles of yoga, such as vinyasa and power yoga. Although I absolutely loved them, I often found myself feeling physically and emotionally drained. I was regularly stressed, had a hard time falling asleep at night, and couldn't meditate for more than 5 minutes at a time. On a hunch, I tried my first yin yoga class— and it was exactly what I needed!

Most of us lead lives that are already yang in nature, meaning we're active and sometimes even overly active. By only practicing yang styles of yoga and leading a busy life, I was burning myself out and not giving myself the chance to slow down and recharge my batteries.

Yin yoga offered me the opportunity to soothe my nervous system, to let go of the need to always be busy, and to learn to truly relax and be in the present moment.

Today, my life and my yoga practice represent a balance between yin and yang. Because of yin yoga, I know how to properly cope with stress, I fall asleep easily, and I genuinely enjoy sitting in meditation. I feel healthier, calmer, and much more flexible—physically and mentally.

This book's intention is to give you the information you need to begin practicing yin yoga at home on your own. Of course, receiving guidance from a teacher in person is tremendously beneficial, but doing yoga at home is a great way to be consistent in your practice. It also gives you the freedom to create your own sequences and the power to learn what your body needs at any given moment.

I hope this book brings you the gift of physical, mental, and emotional health. Most of all, I hope it inspires you to take the first step toward creating more balance in your life.

Kassandra Reinhardt

Yin yoga is a practice of *self-love* and *self-acceptance*

About yin yoga

Within this chapter you'll learn yin yoga philosophies, principles, and techniques that can help you prepare your mind, body, and physical space for a safe and mindful yin yoga experience.

What is yin yoga?

When you hear the word "yoga," you might think of such styles as ashtanga, which is physically demanding and requires extreme focus, or bikram (often referred to as "hot yoga"), which is performed in heated rooms and results in a whole lot of sweat. But yin yoga is different.

The practice

In ancient Chinese philosophy, yin and yang describe how seemingly opposite forces are connected and can help bring balance. This belief also applies to the practice of yoga.

A different style Yin and yang yoga styles move energy throughout the body and help improve physical, mental, and emotional well-being. But yin yoga offers two components that yang yoga lacks: a focus on stillness and an emphasis on longer, deeper stretching of the tissues that surround your body's moving parts. While most yang styles move quickly and focus on muscle tissues, yin yoga moves slowly and stretches more deeply into the body.

A deeper stretch While most forms of yoga focus on building muscle strength and increasing flexibility, yin yoga centers on stretching deeper connective tissues, such as ligaments, tendons, and deep fascia—the tissue that surrounds muscles. This deeper connection is why yin yoga is often called "yoga of the joints."

A passive practice Because you perform yin yoga while sitting or lying down in a passive manner, gravity plays a role in developing a deeper stretch while enabling you to hold poses for longer periods of time. In yin yoga, instead of contracting your muscles to build strength or elevating your heart rate to build stamina, you're encouraged to relax and surrender to gravity.

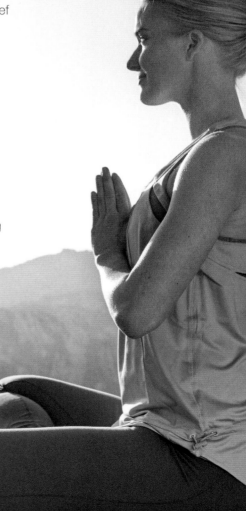

The principles

Sarah Powers, a pioneer of yin yoga, defined three universally acknowledged principles for every practice that together form the basis for practicing yin yoga safely and effectively.

Find your edge Finding your edge—knowing when to stop during a pose—helps create the essential balance between no sensation and too much sensation in the body. You can learn your edge by stopping at a point during a pose where you feel intense sensations. If you go beyond that point, you risk injury.

Be still Once you find your edge, you remain still. Paying attention to your tendency to fidget, move, or mentally distract yourself is the purpose of being still. By achieving a meditative state, you're better able to listen to your body and honor your limits. Being still is critical to your yin yoga practice.

Hold the pose You'll gain the most from your yin yoga practice by holding a pose. While beginning practitioners might start with a 1- to 3-minute hold time, more experienced students might hold asanas anywhere from 5 to 10 minutes.

Ancient origins— modern practice

Yin yoga blends teachings from two different lineages: traditional Indian hatha yoga and the Chinese Taoist yin yang philosophy. Each asana— Sanskrit for "manner of sitting"— is derived from hatha yoga, but the process of holding poses for an extended period of time is rooted in Chinese Taoist practices.

Today, yin yoga serves as an antidote to your often stress-filled and busy life, which is typically yang in nature. Too much yang activity can cause an imbalance on physical, emotional, and mental levels. While you never want to be completely yin, true health and well-being come from the practice of balancing the yin and the yang, the passive and the active, and the calming and the stimulating.

Why do yin yoga?

Yin yoga targets your physical, mental, and emotional concerns through deep stretching and breathing. However, unlike most yang styles of yoga—which typically focuses on stretching muscles and emphasize shorter hold times—yin yoga reaches deeper into your body and mind.

Physical benefits

Your physical body will benefit most from practicing yin yoga because it touches every element of your musculoskeletal system. Yin yoga focuses on your fascia—tissue around muscles and organs—so you should feel improved health on the inside, which should improve how you feel on the outside.

Improved joint health The primary physical benefit of yin yoga is strengthening the connective tissues in your joints. They're strengthened through steady, sustained stretching. By applying stress to your joints through stretching, yin yoga helps open and lubricate tight joints.

Increased mobility As you age, you start losing joint mobility. It's thus essential to keep your hip, lower back, and pelvic areas healthy and flexible so you can remain mobile. Yin yoga can free up those areas to increase range of motion and improve flexibility in these zones, making movement and mobility freer and easier.

Better organ function Yin yoga is thought to benefit your heart and lungs through increased blood flow and deeper breathing. Many asanas also include moves that compress and decompress your abdomen, which is believed to help stimulate your digestive system and promote healthier kidney and intestine functions.

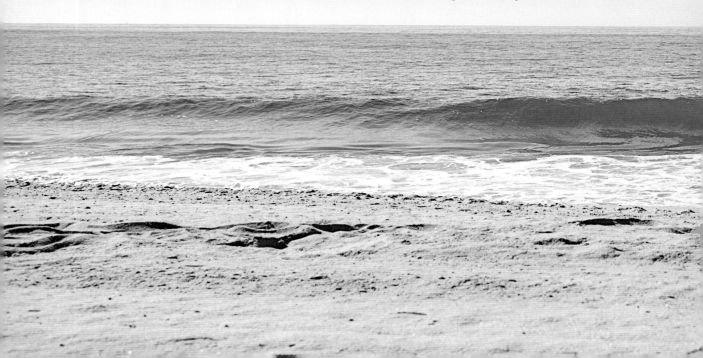

Mental and emotional benefits

In addition to physical benefits, like improved digestion, better mobility, and cardiovascular health, practicing yin yoga on a regular basis might alleviate feelings of stress and anxiety, help improve your sleep, and have a positive effect on your mental and emotional states.

Stillness of the mind Yin yoga has a deeply meditative quality that allows you to quiet down an overactive mind and tune in to your immediate surroundings. When you remove external stimuli and surrender to the present moment, you can enter into a meditative state and let go of mental clutter to achieve a greater sense of inner peace and calm.

Relief from stress Remaining in a high-alert state might cause health issues, including high blood pressure and heart problems. Certain asanas might help lower blood pressure and slow down your heart rate to create a greater sense of calm.

Emotional healing When your body is still and your mind is silent, certain feelings—such as sadness, excitement, or anger—might arise either during or shortly after practice. Experiencing these emotions is perfectly normal and a healthy effect; your task is simply to observe them as they move through you.

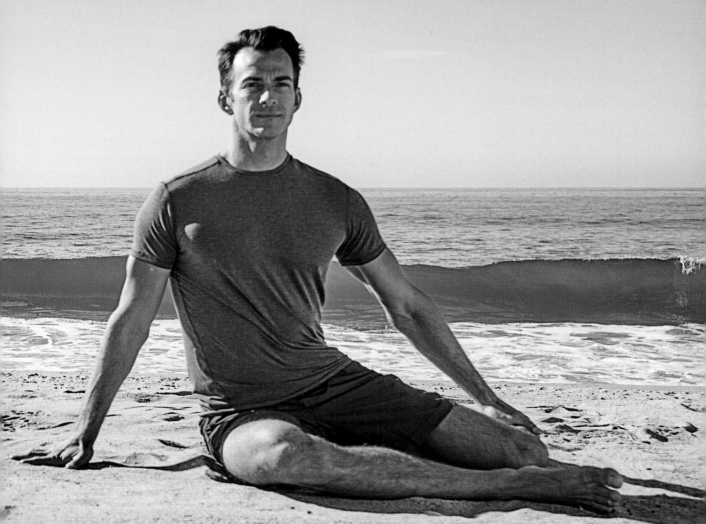

What are chakras?

According to ancient Eastern traditions, chakras (Sanskrit for "wheels" or "discs") are energy points within your spiritual body through which *prana*—your life force or life energy—travels.

How chakras work

Yin yoga encompasses more than just poses and breathing exercises for your physical body. It might also have a positive impact on your energetic body by clearing your chakras. It's thought that these energy centers allow for the flow of *prana* through your body, helping to promote physical, mental, and emotional well-being.

The tenets of this ancient philosophy say that when your chakras are blocked, you might experience physical maladies, such as muscle tightness or joint stiffness, or emotional manifestations, such as recurring fears or negative emotions. It's believed that practicing yin yoga can help clear chakras of energetic blockages and restore their balance.

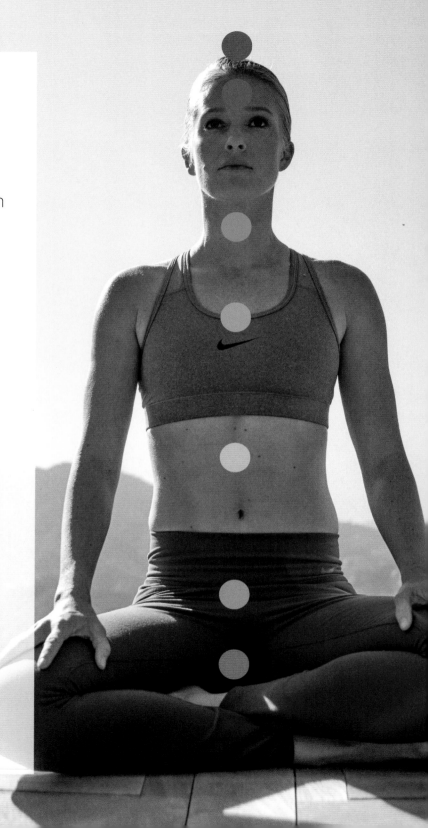

The seven chakras and their bijas

Repeating aloud a mantra—called a *bija*, which means "seed" in Sanskrit—can unlock each chakra's energy. A *bija* is a sound that should be verbalized and sustained for the length of an exhale. Once the exhale is complete, breathe in and repeat the *bija* for the next exhale.

Chakra	Governs	When balanced	Bijas and asanas
Crown (*sahasrara* in Sanskrit)	Your connection to the universe and is associated with spirituality and enlightenment	You'll feel more connected and more blissful	Bija mantra: OM (or silence) Suggested asanas: any breathing technique, Seated meditation, or Corpse
Third eye (*ajna* in Sanskrit)	Your mind and inner wisdom and is associated with insight, psychic awareness, and imagination	You'll feel better able to tap into your intuition more deeply and see the bigger picture more easily	Bija mantra: OM Suggested asana: Child's pose
Throat (*vishuddha* in Sanskrit)	Your ability to communicate with others and speak the truth and is associated with self-expression, discernment, and honesty	You'll feel more free to speak what's on your mind and in your heart while also learning to be a better listener	Bija mantra: HAM Suggested asana: Neck release
Heart (*anahata* in Sanskrit)	Your ability to relate and empathize with others and is associated with love, gratitude, and forgiveness	You'll feel better able to express love unconditionally and feel more compassion for all beings	Bija mantra: YAM Suggested asana: Supported fish
Solar plexus (*manipura* in Sanskrit)	Your relationship with yourself and is associated with self-esteem, willpower, and determination	You'll feel more confident, worthy of respect, and capable	Bija mantra: RAM Suggested asana: Lying spinal twist
Sacral (*svadhisthana* in Sanskrit)	Your relationships and emotions and is associated with sexuality and creativity	You'll feel more comfortable with your sexuality, more inspired, and more deeply connected to others	Bija mantra: VAM Suggested asana: Any dragon asana
Root (*muladhara* in Sanskrit)	Your ties to your culture and the physical world and is associated with safety, self-preservation, and survival	You'll feel more grounded, abundant, and secure	Bija mantra: LAM Suggested asanas: Deer or Squat

What are meridians?

In Chinese medicine, energy called *Qi* (pronounced "chee") flows through you in pathways called meridians. When healthy and clear, these pathways might increase longevity and support the proper function of your organs.

How meridians work

Meridians can be described as channels or pathways that control the flow of energy to and from various points in your body. They're not vessels in the physiological sense; they're more akin to energy paths that when clear might promote the efficient flow of energy through your body.

Liver	Gall bladder	Kidney	Bladder	Spleen	Stomach
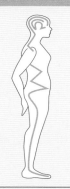	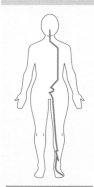	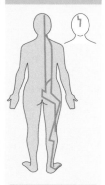	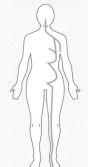	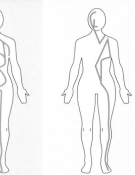	
Associated with: blood flow, tendon and ligament flexibility, and menstrual cycles	**Associated with:** bile and energy for movement and action	**Associated with:** sexual energy and the production of bone marrow	**Associated with:** the removal of liquid waste from the body	**Associated with:** digestion and the flow of nutrients in the body	**Associated with:** digestion and the mental state
When unbalanced: believed to cause stomach pain, back pain, stiffness in the joints, anger, and irritability	**When unbalanced:** believed to cause headaches, eye disorders, insomnia, timidness, and indecisiveness	**When unbalanced:** believed to cause urinary disorders, reproduction issues, back pain, fear, and insecurity	**When unbalanced:** believed to cause back pain, urinary disorders, vision problems, and indecisiveness	**When unbalanced:** believed to cause digestion issues, stomach problems, fatigue, brain fog, and excessive worry	**When unbalanced:** believed to cause digestion issues, stomach pain, excessive worry, and anxiety
Asana to help return you to balance: Straddle	**Asana to help return you to balance:** Banana	**Asana to help return you to balance:** Butterfly	**Asana to help return you to balance:** Caterpillar	**Asana to help return you to balance:** Saddle	**Asana to help return you to balance:** Twisted dragon

The 12 meridians and their asanas

It's believed that stress, difficulty processing emotions, and improper diet can block the meridians and immobilize the *Qi* flow in your body, causing physical problems or disease. The principles of this philosophy suggest that yin yoga might be ideal for helping to open up these blocked meridians, allowing *Qi* to more freely flow throughout your body, and bringing you more internal and external strength.

Practicing the asanas in this book on a regular basis might help stimulate the meridians and allow your *Qi* to freely flow, nourishing your organs and replenishing your energy levels. By improving the health of your connective tissues and calming your mind and emotions through practice, you can allow *Qi* to flow more openly through your meridians. Whenever you feel out of balance, practicing yin yoga might unblock your meridians.

Heart	Small intestine	Lung	Large intestine	Pericardium	Triple burner
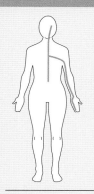	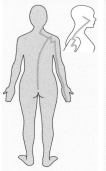 	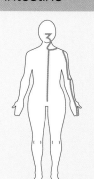	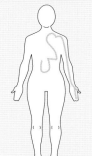	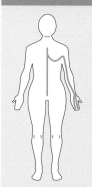	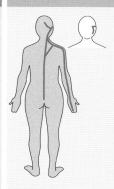
Associated with: distributing blood to organs and governing emotions	**Associated with:** the separation of nutrients to be absorbed and eliminated	**Associated with:** the regulation of breath and the intake of energy	**Associated with:** the elimination of waste and the reabsorption of water	**Associated with:** the removal of excess energy and the protection of the heart	**Associated with:** the regulation of metabolism
When unbalanced: believed to cause chest pain, heart palpitations, sleep problems, anxiety, and depression	**When unbalanced:** believed to cause digestion issues, poor circulation, lower abdomen pain, and poor mental clarity	**When unbalanced:** believed to cause respiratory problems, throat and nose issues, sadness, and grief	**When unbalanced:** believed to cause constipation, sore throat, abdominal pain, worry, and difficulty letting go	**When unbalanced:** believed to cause heart problems, negative sexual feelings, and difficulty expressing emotions	**When unbalanced:** believed to cause appetite dysfunction, ear and throat problems, and emotional instability
Asana to help return you to balance: Sphinx	**Asana to help return you to balance:** Bowtie	**Asana to help return you to balance:** Melting heart	**Asana to help return you to balance:** Lying chest opener	**Asana to help return you to balance:** Wrist extensor stretch	**Asana to help return you to balance:** Eagle arms

Breathing techniques

Pranayama—the Sanskrit word for breathing exercises and controls—can help you balance your energy levels, facilitate a meditative state, and support your body during your yin yoga practice. Practicing *pranayama* will help you slow down and deepen your breathing.

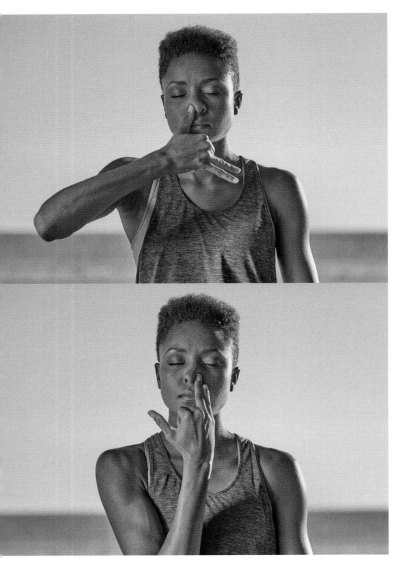

Alternate nostril breath

Perform the alternate nostril breath—called *nadi shodan* in Sanskrit—before practicing an asana as opposed to during an asana. It can balance your energy levels and calm you down when you're overactive and stressed. You can even use this technique when not practicing yin yoga.

1 Sit in a cross-legged position, with your hands resting on your thighs.

2 Lift your right hand up and bend your index and middle fingers toward your palm, bringing your right thumb to your right nostril and pressing to seal it shut.

3 Deeply inhale through your left nostril for a count of 4, 5, or 6.

4 Seal off your left nostril with your right ring finger and release your right nostril.

5 Exhale through your right nostril for the same count of 4, 5, or 6.

6 Deeply inhale through your right nostril for a count of 4, 5, or 6.

7 Seal off your right nostril with your right thumb and release your left nostril.

8 Exhale through your left nostril for the same count of 4, 5, or 6 to complete one round. Repeat these steps for 5 to 10 more rounds.

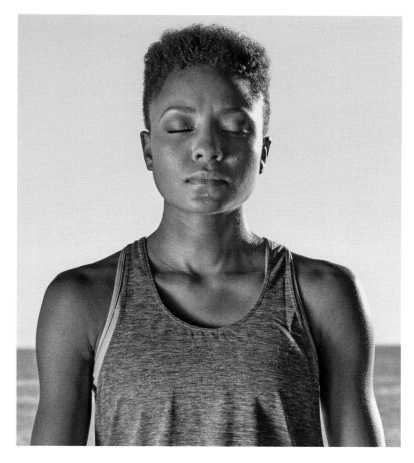

Ocean breath

The ocean breath—called *ujjayi* in Sanskrit—is a breathing exercise you can do while performing yin yoga asanas. As you practice this technique, imagine you're trying to fog up a mirror with your breath while keeping your mouth closed, breathing only through your nostrils. You should make a slight constriction at the back of your throat, which should produce a soft sound similar to that of an ocean.

1 With a slight throat constriction, inhale through your nose for a count of 4, 5, or 6.

2 Pause at the top of the inhale for a count of 1.

3 With a slight throat constriction, exhale through your nose for a count of 4, 5, or 6.

4 Pause at the end of the exhale for a count of 1 to complete one round. Repeat these steps for 5 to 10 rounds.

Humming bee breath

Performing humming bee breath—called *bhramari* in Sanskrit— is best done before practicing an asana. This simple breathing exercise can help calm your nerves and quiet a busy mind.

1 Sit in a cross-legged position, with your hands resting on your thighs.

2 Press your index fingers to the cartilage between your cheek and ear to block outside noise, keeping your elbows lifted.

3 Inhale a deep breath through your nose.

4 Exhale through your nose while making a long "mmmmm" sound aloud—like a bee buzzing— to complete one round. Repeat these steps for 3 to 5 rounds.

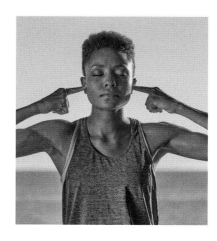

What do you need?

Props are essential components of a yin yoga practice and allow you to perform yin asanas more safely and effectively. The most commonly used yin yoga props discussed here are featured throughout this book.

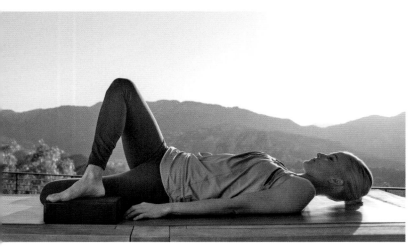

Blocks

Blocks are used to fill the gaps between your body and the ground and to provide support for your body during more challenging poses.

What to buy: Blocks come in wood, cork, foam, and bamboo, giving you several different options for comfort and budget. It's best to have two blocks on hand for your yin yoga practice. You can also use large—but firm—pillows.

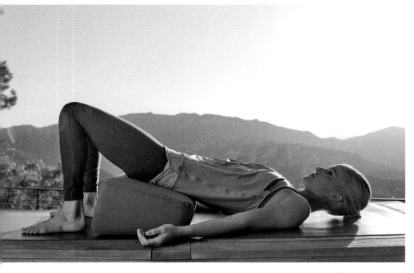

Bolsters

Bolsters are large yoga pillows that are useful for providing support during more difficult positions. Bolsters provide you with a more stable surface that you can lie back on or use to prop yourself up comfortably, which will help you hold poses for extended periods of time.

What to buy: Choose a large rectangular or cylindrical bolster that's roughly the length of your spine. You can also use a dense couch cushion or pillow.

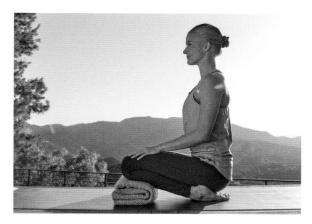

Yoga blankets

Yoga blankets provide extra padding for your hands and knees, especially if you have a thinner mat. They also can be used to provide comfort and support to your legs when you're sitting cross-legged and need to elevate your hips.

What to buy: Cotton is your best bet, but you can also use thick blankets you already own.

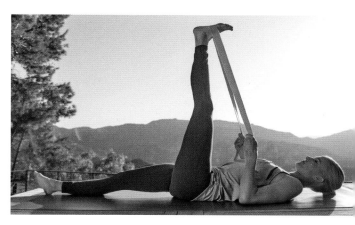

Straps

Straps will help you extend your reach if you have limited flexibility. They'll also help you gain stability and perform reclining asanas more efficiently.

What to buy: Most yoga straps are between 6 (1.75m) and 10 feet (3m) long. Choose one that feels comfortable between your hands. You can also use a belt or a length of soft rope.

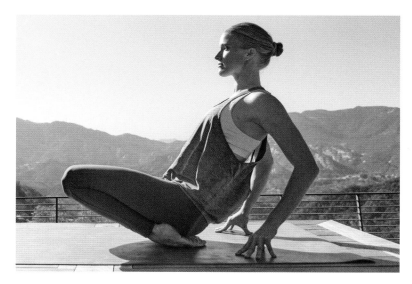

Mats

A yoga mat is used to provide comfort and keep your body off the surface below you. It will also help you maintain balance.

What to buy: Consider thickness when buying a yoga mat. Standard mats are usually ⅛-inch (3 mm) thick, but if you have sensitive joints, a mat that's ¼-inch (6mm) thick will provide additional support. If you don't have a mat, use a blanket.

How do you practice?

Reaping the full benefits of yin yoga requires you to hold poses for extended periods of time. This section will help ensure that your body and mind are prepared for a complete yin experience.

How and when to practice

Make the most of your yin yoga practice by creating an environment in which you have the physical space and the time to have an effective and consistent yin yoga experience.

Find a quiet, peaceful space
Choose one that's free of distractions. Maintaining a home yoga practice means making the time you spend on your mat feel like a retreat from the stresses of everyday life. Your peaceful space doesn't have to be fancy nor does it need to be indoors, but you should feel safe and protected from distractions— electronic or otherwise.

Set the mood You can set the mood for a more meditative atmosphere by playing soft ambient music in the background, lighting a few candles, or using essential oils.

Stage your props To prevent the need to pause after you've started, have all the necessary props required for that day's asanas laid out around you before you begin.

Practice with cold muscles
Practicing when your muscles are cold helps to emphasize the strengthening and lengthening of the connective tissues,

as opposed to the muscles. This means you don't need to perform any warmups.

Refrain from eating Avoid eating a meal right before practice. Give your body a few hours to digest food before practice so you'll feel comfortable in the poses.

Start your experience slowly
If you're new to yin yoga, start by practicing once or twice a week and increase that number if your body allows it, ensuring to take at least one full day's rest every week. And make sure you start each practice with the seated meditation (see page 24).

Using this book

This book is made up of asanas and sequences. Asanas are individual poses, and sequences are a series of asanas targeting a specific goal.

The asanas Each asana includes step-by-step instructions for effectively performing the pose. Read through every step before attempting a pose, including any modifications. Listen to your body and change the hold times depending on how you feel. Be sure to note any physical concerns or limitations included with each asana so you can perform each one safely.

The asana's effects

Step-by-step instructions

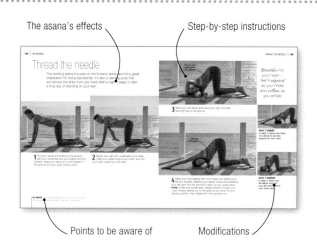

Points to be aware of

Modifications

Practice early or late An early morning session can awaken your body and mind for the day ahead. It can also help loosen up joints that are stiff from a long night of sleep. A session just before bedtime can place your mind and body in a restful state and prepare you for a better night of sleep. Practice yin yoga when it feels right for you.

Plan ahead Set time aside for your practice—whether every day or every other day. Remember that you'll be holding poses for long periods of time, so you won't be doing too many asanas during a 30-minute session. And remember to include time for any breathing exercises you might want to do.

End every session in Corpse pose Resting in Corpse pose for a few minutes at the end of your practice will give your mind and body an opportunity to fully integrate the work you've done during the practice.

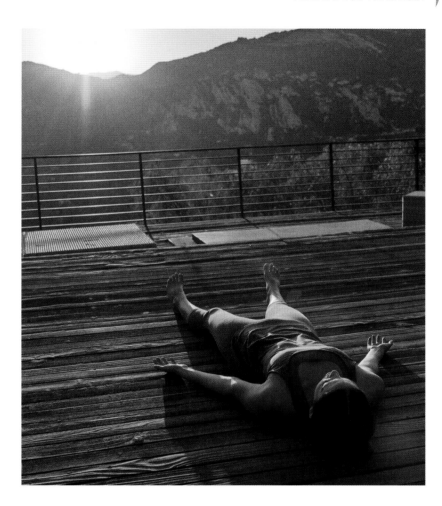

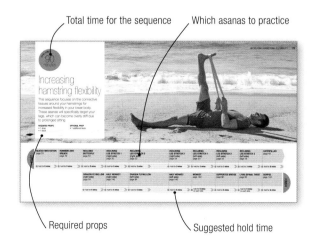

Total time for the sequence

Which asanas to practice

Required props

Suggested hold time

The sequences In addition to individual asanas, there are 20 sequences—which group specific asanas together—with total hold times ranging from 30 to 90 minutes. Before starting a selected sequence, read through all the asanas and ensure you have all needed props nearby. You can modify sequences to suit your needs by changing the hold times of the asanas, adding or removing meditations or breathing techniques, or performing the "Make it easier" or "Make it harder" options for an asana.

Seated meditation

Begin your yin yoga practice with the seated meditation, which will help ease you into a meditative state before practicing the poses in this book. Finding a restful, meditative state is as easy as following a few steps — with the goal being to gradually lengthen the spaces between thoughts.

How to meditate

Meditation is a simple process, but the benefits are immeasurable. Before you begin, try to find a peaceful, quiet location that's free of any distractions.

1 Sit in a comfortable seated position. Place your hands on your thighs or knees, straighten your back, and extend the crown of your head upward.

2 Close your eyes and visualize yourself in a peaceful place. Focus on the sensations you might feel — such as a light breeze on your face or the sound of running water — as if you were there.

3 Imagine your body being surrounded by a warm, radiant white light.

4 Inhale slow, steady breaths through your nose and imagine yourself breathing in the light.

5 Allow your body and mind to relax as you exhale slowly through your nose. Remain in this position for as long as desired.

Helpful hints

- If you notice discomfort in your hips or lower back, sit on a block or a folded blanket for support.

- If you feel your muscles tightening up, bring your awareness back to your breathing and focus on relaxing your muscles with every exhale.

- If you're struggling with a recurring negative thought or emotion, imagine inhaling a calm feeling and expelling the negative thought or emotion with each exhale.

- If you want to achieve an even deeper level of relaxation, internally repeat a *bija* (mantra) as you inhale deeply through your nose and again for the duration of your exhale.

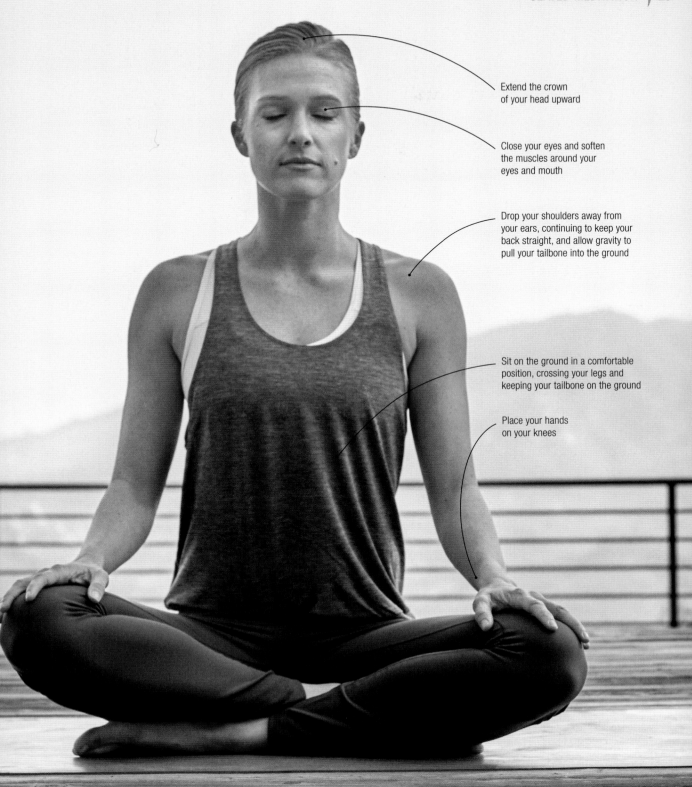

Extend the crown
of your head upward

Close your eyes and soften
the muscles around your
eyes and mouth

Drop your shoulders away from
your ears, continuing to keep your
back straight, and allow gravity to
pull your tailbone into the ground

Sit on the ground in a comfortable
position, crossing your legs and
keeping your tailbone on the ground

Place your hands
on your knees

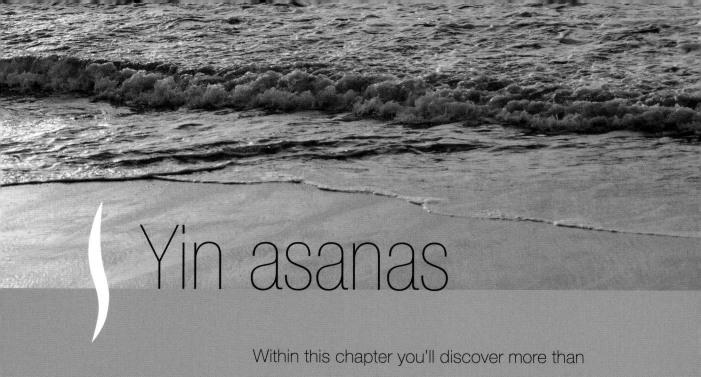

Yin asanas

Within this chapter you'll discover more than 50 yoga poses—each designed to be held for an extended period. These asanas were created with one goal: to offer life-changing impacts on your body *and* your mind.

Square

This asana stretches your lower back, helps reinforce outer hip rotation (which can help alleviate knee strain), and might promote healthy digestion by compressing your stomach.

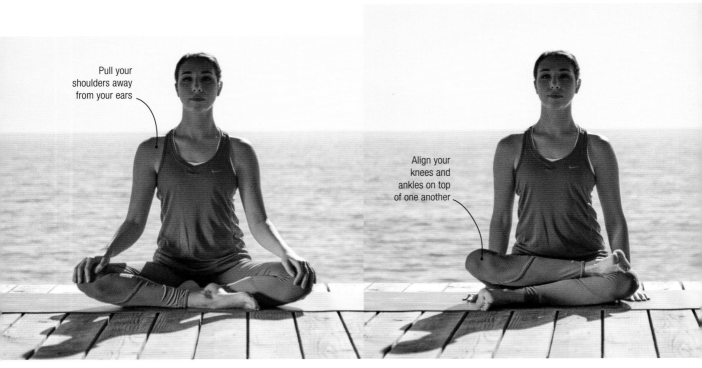

Pull your shoulders away from your ears

Align your knees and ankles on top of one another

1 Sit on the ground in a comfortable position, crossing your legs and keeping your tailbone on the ground. Put your hands on your knees and extend the crown of your head upward.

2 Place your right foot on your left knee and tuck your left foot under your right knee. Flex your feet so your toes point toward your knees.

BE AWARE If you have sciatica or knee pain or have ever suffered lower-back or knee injuries, you should avoid this pose because it could aggravate those conditions.

Allow any *distractions*
to drift into the background—
stay present

Keep your neck
and back straight
to avoid hunching

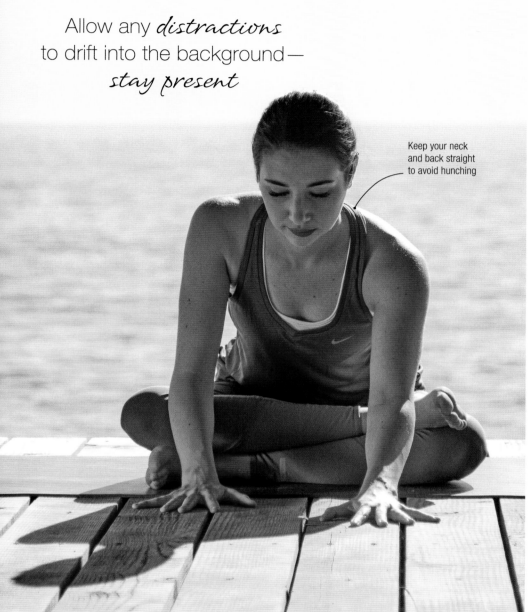

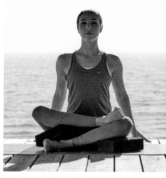

MAKE IT EASIER
In step 2, place
blocks under
your knees and
put your hands
behind you.

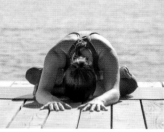

MAKE IT HARDER
In step 3, place
your hands farther
away from your
body and rest
your forehead
and forearms
on the ground.

3 Lean forward from your hips and slide your hands forward
until you find your edge, but don't go all the way to the ground.
Hold. Inhale and exhale slow, steady breaths through your nose.
Slowly reverse out of the pose.

Reclining leg stretch 1

This asana opens up your entire leg—from hamstring to ankle— providing a full lower-body stretch without putting excess stress on your lower back. You'll need a strap for this pose.

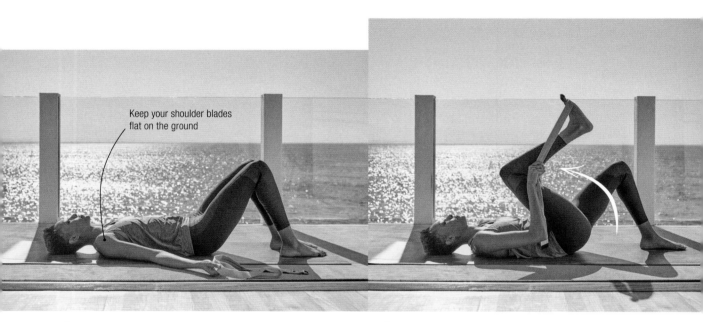

Keep your shoulder blades flat on the ground

1 Lie on your back and bend your knees, keeping your feet flat on the ground. Relax your arms at your sides and hold the strap in your right hand.

2 Transfer one end of the strap to your left hand and bring your right knee toward your chest. Slip the strap around the ball of your right foot.

BE AWARE If you've ever suffered hamstring injuries or tears, you should avoid this pose or use caution by keeping your extended leg slightly bent at your knee.

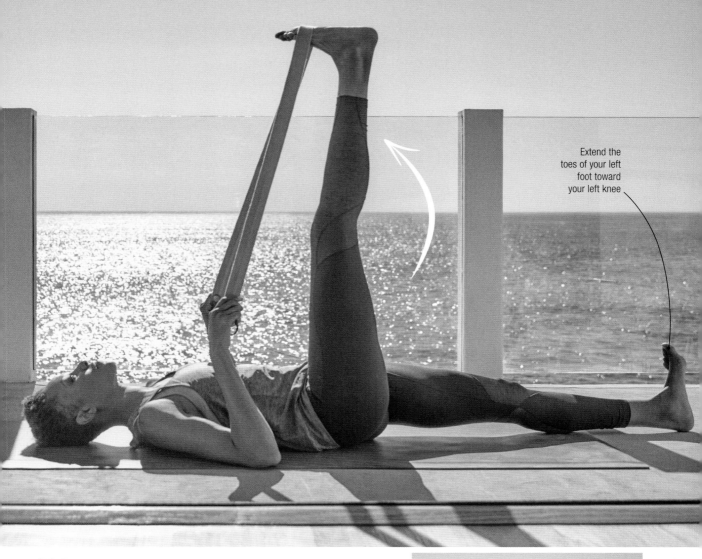

Extend the
toes of your left
foot toward
your left knee

3 Extend your right leg upward while extending your left leg until it's flat on the ground. Pull your shoulders toward the ground and lightly pull on the strap to bring your right foot closer to your head without bending your knee. **Hold.** Inhale and exhale slow, steady breaths through your nose. Slowly reverse out of the pose as you return to your starting position, then repeat with the opposite leg.

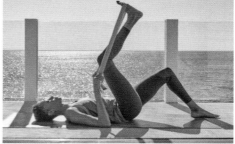

MAKE IT EASIER
In step 3, keep both knees slightly bent.

Reclining leg stretch 2

This asana cultivates deep flexibility in your inner groin and hamstrings while allowing your upper back to relax. It can also help restore energy to your body. You'll need a strap for this pose.

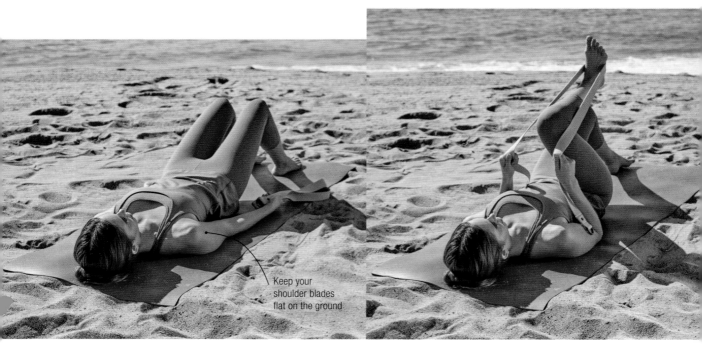

Keep your shoulder blades flat on the ground

1 Lie on your back and bend your knees, keeping your feet flat on the ground. Relax your arms at your sides and hold the strap in your right hand.

2 Transfer one end of the strap to your left hand and bring your right knee toward your chest. Slip the strap around the ball of your right foot.

BE AWARE If you feel pain in your neck or upper back, you can place a blanket or pillow under your head to help your neck and upper back remain comfortable.

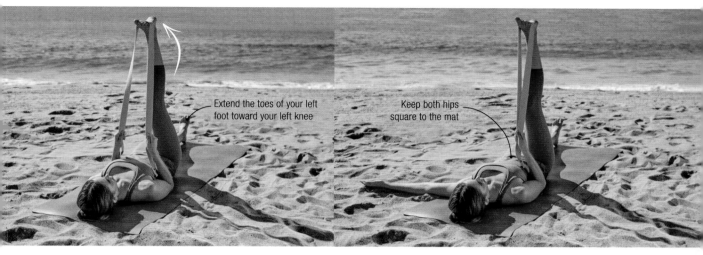

Extend the toes of your left foot toward your left knee

Keep both hips square to the mat

3 Extend your right leg upward while extending your left leg until it's flat on the ground. Pull your shoulders toward the ground and lightly pull the strap to bring your right leg closer to your head without bending your knee.

4 Transfer both ends of the strap to your right hand and extend your left arm so it's perpendicular to your body. Keep your left arm and your shoulder blades flat on the ground.

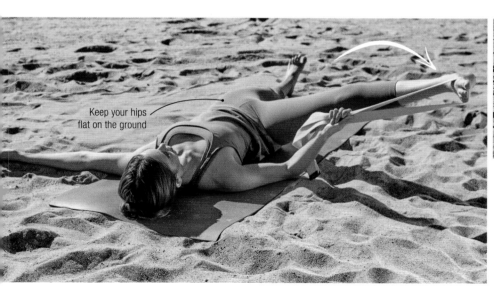

Keep your hips flat on the ground

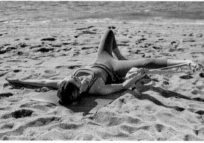

MAKE IT EASIER
In step 5, bend your left knee, but keep your left foot flat on the ground. You can also place a bolster under your right thigh.

5 Keep your right leg fully extended as you lightly pull your right leg so it's almost parallel to your left arm. **Hold.** Inhale and exhale slow, steady breaths through your nose. Slowly reverse out of the pose as you return to your starting position, then repeat with the opposite leg.

Reclining leg stretch 3

This twisting asana—which can stretch your chest and help relieve lower-back pain—encourages healthy digestion and offers a deep leg stretch. You'll need a strap for this pose.

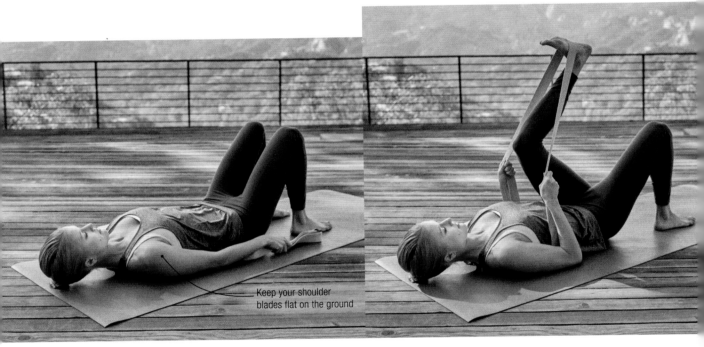

Keep your shoulder blades flat on the ground

1 Lie on your back and bend your knees, keeping your feet flat on the ground. Relax your arms at your sides and hold a strap in your right hand.

2 Transfer one end of the strap to your left hand and bring your left knee toward your chest. Slip the strap around the ball of your left foot.

BE AWARE If you've suffered slipped or herniated discs, you should avoid this pose because it could aggravate those conditions.

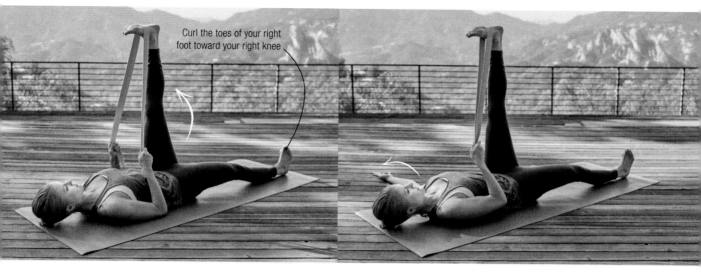

Curl the toes of your right foot toward your right knee

3 Extend your left leg upward while extending your right leg until it's flat on the ground. Continue to keep your head, shoulder blades, and right heel flat on the ground.

4 Transfer both ends of the strap to your right hand. Extend your left arm until it's perpendicular to your body, keeping it flat on the ground, with your left palm facing up.

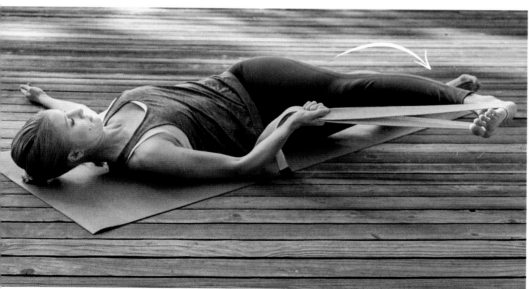

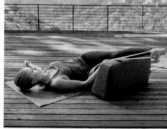

MAKE IT EASIER
In step 5, support your twisting leg with a block or a bolster.

5 Cross your left leg over your right leg, making your left leg parallel to your left arm. **Hold.** Inhale and exhale slow, steady breaths through your nose. Slowly reverse out of the pose as you return to your starting position, then repeat with the opposite leg.

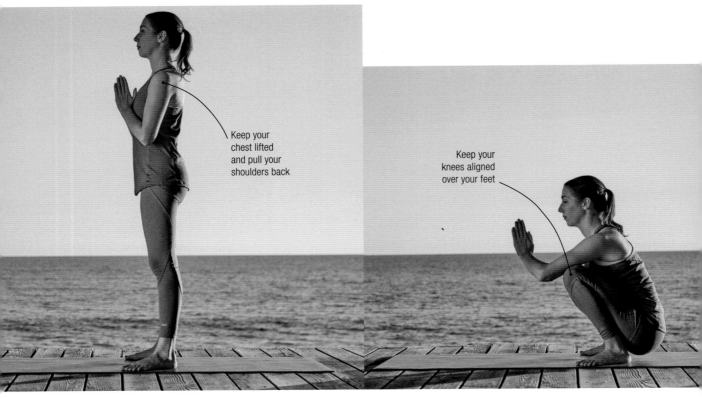

Keep your chest lifted and pull your shoulders back

Keep your knees aligned over your feet

1 Stand with your feet hip-width distance apart. Turn your feet out so your toes point toward the top corners of the mat and put your hands in a praying position at your heart.

2 Bend your knees to lower your hips toward the ground. Your hips should hover off the ground and your feet should remain flat on the ground.

Squat

This soothing and stabilizing asana helps with outer hip rotation and opens up your lower back. Staying in a low position can help you attain the grounded feelings—physically and mentally—you need for balance in your life.

BE AWARE Although this asana can strengthen your ankles, if you've ever suffered any kind of ankle injury, use caution during this pose or perform the Reclined child's pose (page 120) instead.

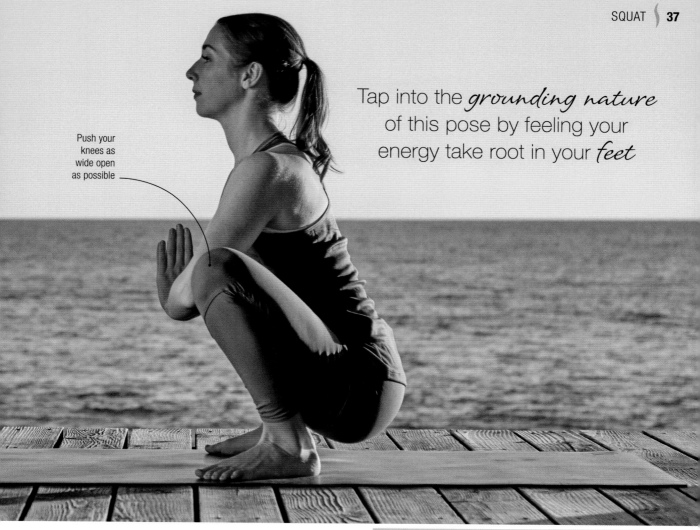

Push your knees as wide open as possible

Tap into the *grounding nature* of this pose by feeling your energy take root in your *feet*

3 Rest your elbows on the inside of your thighs and use your arms to press your knees open. Extend the crown of your head upward and lengthen your tailbone to elongate your spine. **Hold.** Inhale and exhale slow, steady breaths through your nose. Slowly reverse out of the pose.

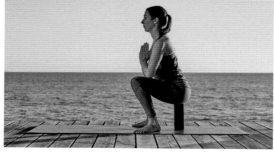

MAKE IT EASIER
In step 2, place a block under your hips for elevation. You can also place a rolled-up blanket under your heels if they're lifting off the ground.

Toe squat

This asana targets your lower legs—an area often neglected by traditional exercise. Having flexible feet will help you maintain a strong foundation for balance and agility.

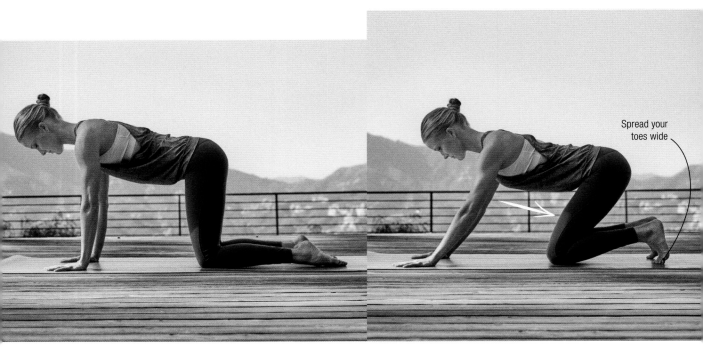

Spread your toes wide

1 Put your hands and knees flat on the ground, pointing your fingers forward. Keep your spine and neck parallel to the ground and your eyes looking down.

2 Flex your feet and curl your toes toward your knees, keeping your toes flat on the ground. Shift your body back to center your hips over your heels, continuing to align your neck and back.

BE AWARE While this asana stretches the toes and soles of your feet, if you have weak knees or ankles, you might find this pose uncomfortable or difficult to hold.

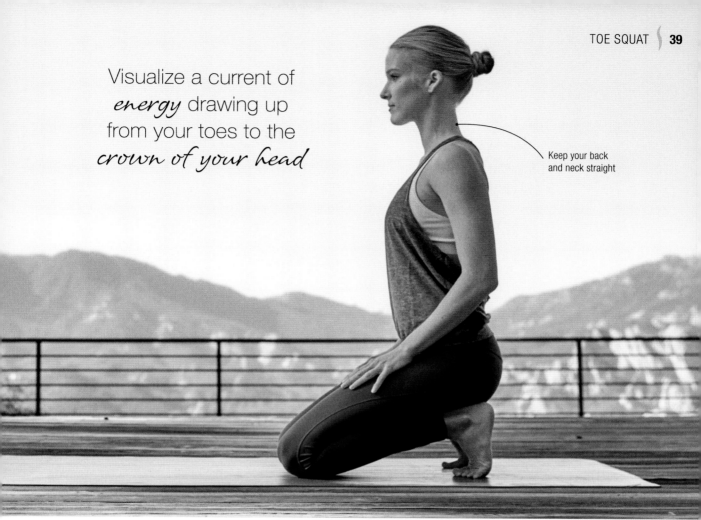

Visualize a current of *energy* drawing up from your toes to the *crown of your head*

Keep your back and neck straight

3 Continue to shift your hips back to rest them on your heels. Place your palms on your thighs. **Hold.** Inhale and exhale slow, steady breaths through your nose. Slowly reverse out of the pose.

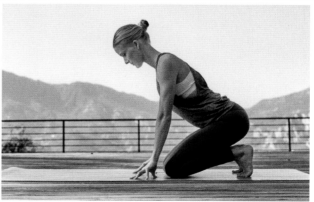

MAKE IT EASIER
In step 3, keep your hips slightly elevated and put your hands on the ground out in front of you, using only your fingers for support.

IT band stretch

Runners will appreciate this hip-opening asana that targets the legs—
from your hips to your knees. In this area are your iliotibial (IT) bands—
the connective tissues that extend from your pelvic bone to your
shinbone—which are difficult to target and thus easy to neglect.

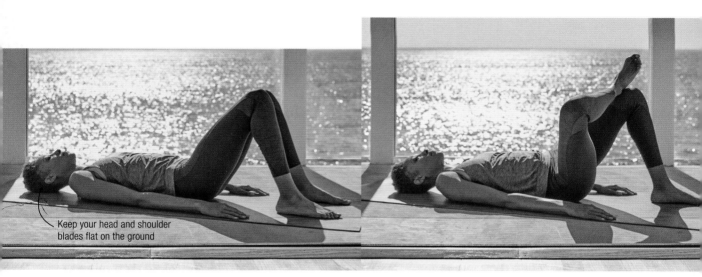

Keep your head and shoulder
blades flat on the ground

1 Lie on your back and bend your knees,
relaxing your arms at your sides and
keeping your feet and hands flat on the
ground. Relax your neck and look straight
up toward the sky.

2 Slowly raise your right foot over your left
knee and rest your right ankle just above
your left knee. Extend your right toes upward
to relieve tension on your right knee and gently
push your right knee away from your body.

BE AWARE Although this pose can help with post-workout recovery, use caution if you
have IT band syndrome because overstretching the IT band could aggravate the problem.

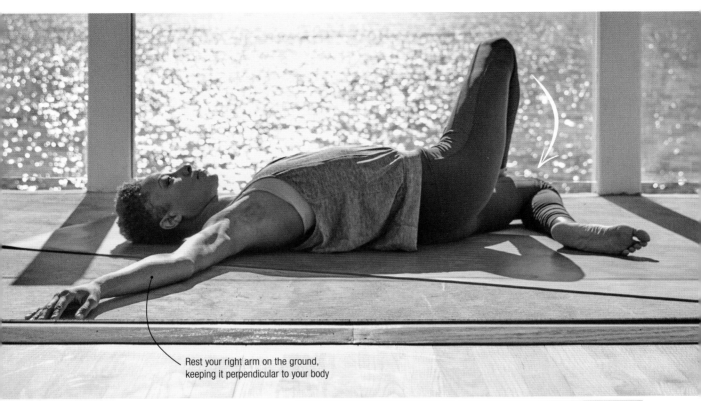

Rest your right arm on the ground, keeping it perpendicular to your body

3 Rotate your hips to lower your left thigh and right foot toward the ground on your left side until your right foot makes contact with the ground. Grab your right ankle with your left hand. **Hold.** Inhale and exhale slow, steady breaths through your nose. Slowly reverse out of the pose as you return to your starting position, then repeat with the opposite leg.

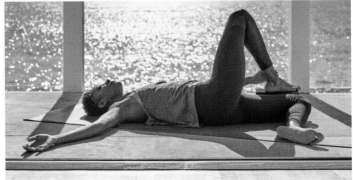

MAKE IT EASIER
In step 3, place a block under the foot of the crossing leg.

Neck release

Neck tension is one of the most common complaints people have. Taking a few minutes to stretch this area can help you release stress and improve your posture.

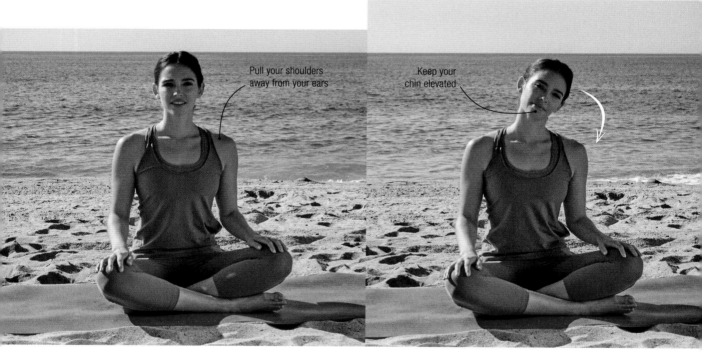

Pull your shoulders away from your ears

Keep your chin elevated

1 Sit on the ground in a comfortable position, crossing your legs and keeping your tailbone on the ground. Put your hands on your knees and extend the crown of your head upward.

2 Drop your left ear toward your left shoulder without letting your chin drop to your chest. Keep your shoulders level and aligned over your hips and let your head become heavy so your neck can relax.

BE AWARE If you've ever suffered a cervical spine injury, you can tilt your head in a different direction or you can avoid this pose entirely.

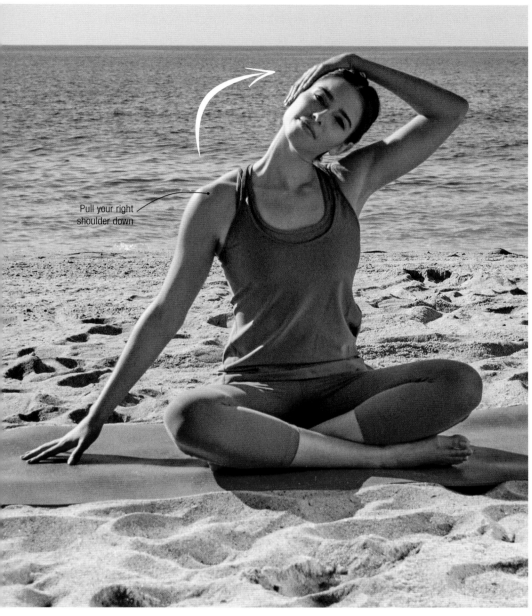

Pull your right shoulder down

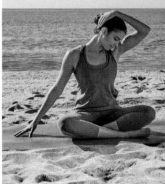

MAKE IT EASIER
In step 3, put your hand behind your right ear and let your chin tilt down toward your left shoulder.

3 Reach your right arm out to your right side, putting your fingertips on the ground, and curl your left hand over your head to place it over your right ear. Pull your head farther away from your right shoulder.
Hold. Inhale and exhale slow, steady breaths through your nose. Slowly reverse out of the pose as you return to your starting position, then repeat with the opposite hand.

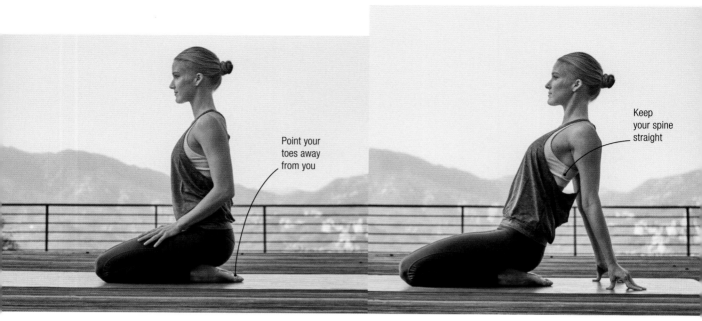

Point your
toes away
from you

Keep
your spine
straight

1 Sit in a kneeling position, allowing your hips
to sit on your heels. Rest your palms on
your thighs and extend the crown of your
head upward.

2 Reach your arms behind you, putting
your fingers on the ground for support
and pointing them away from you as you
shift your weight back onto your feet.

Ankle stretch

If you have problems kneeling or squatting, this asana can help
improve the flexibility in your ankles and allow you to perform those
types of movements more easily.

BE AWARE This is a simple but intense stretch, so if you find this pose uncomfortable
or difficult to hold or if you have inflexible ankles, use a blanket for balance support.

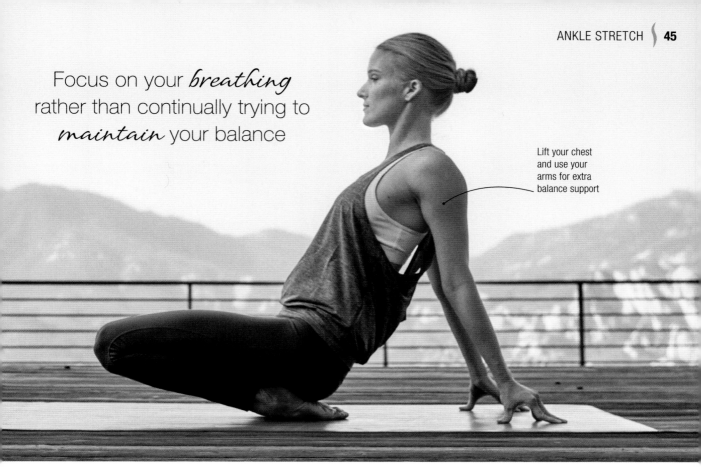

Focus on your *breathing* rather than continually trying to *maintain* your balance

Lift your chest and use your arms for extra balance support

3 Lift your knees and shins off the ground, continuing to use your fingers for support. **Hold.** Inhale and exhale slow, steady breaths through your nose. Slowly reverse out of the pose.

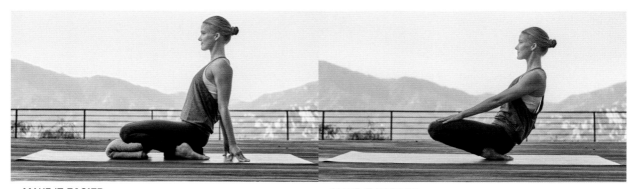

MAKE IT EASIER
In step 3, place a block under your hips and a folded blanket under your knees.

MAKE IT HARDER
In step 3, go deeper into the pose by putting your palms on your knees while still lifting your shins off the ground. Use your core strength to help you stay balanced.

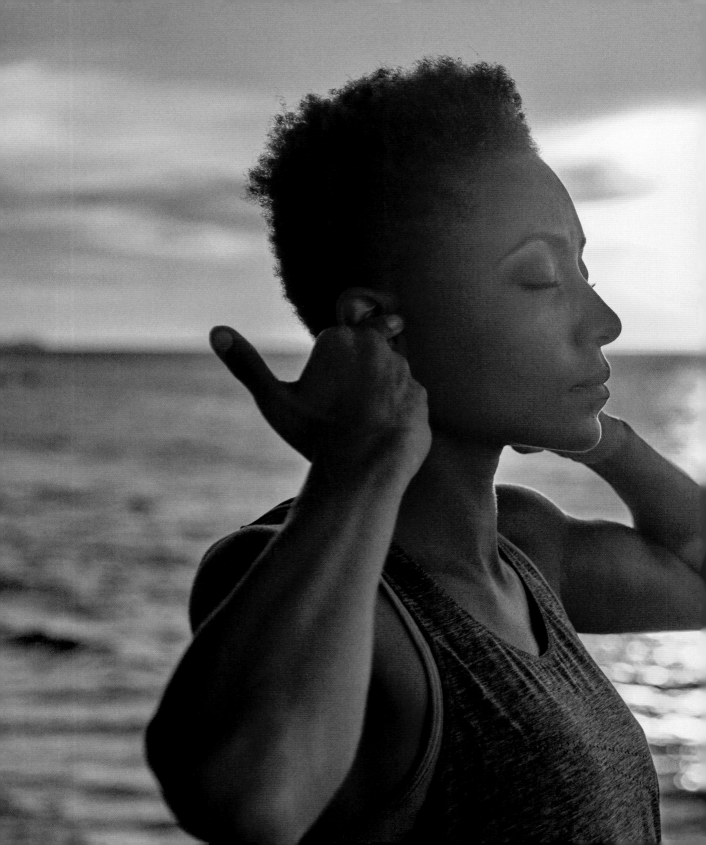

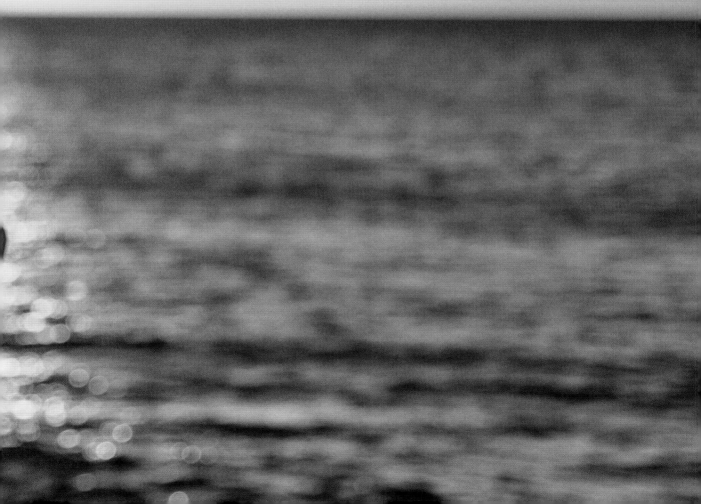
"Yoga is the practice of *quieting the mind*"
Patanjali

Caterpillar

This asana provides a full-body stretch—ideal for relaxation and eliminating stress. It might also help with digestion because the forward fold compresses your stomach.

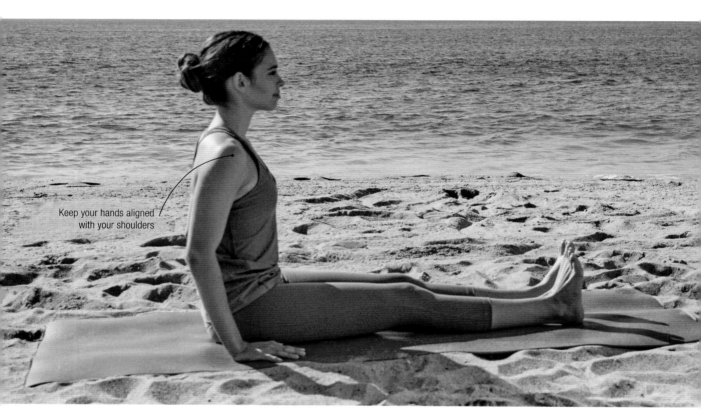

Keep your hands aligned with your shoulders

1 Sit up tall, stretching your legs out in front of you and placing your hands on the ground at your sides. Keep your tailbone on the ground and extend the crown of your head upward.

BE AWARE Because this asana can stretch the muscles around your spine, if you have sciatica pain, performing this pose could aggravate that condition.

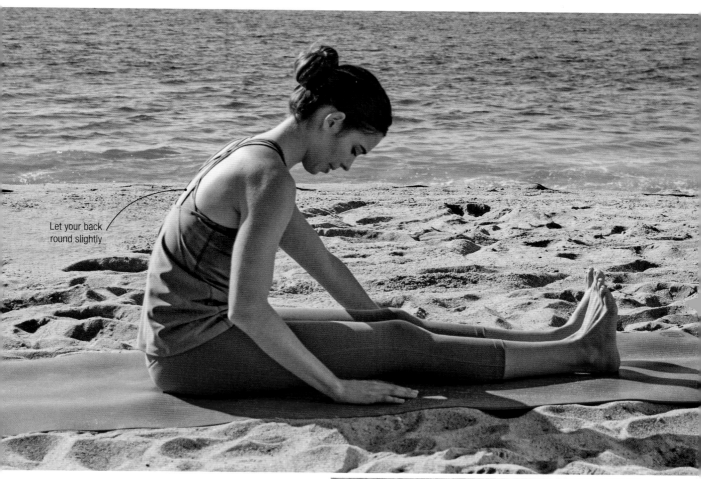

Let your back round slightly

2 Walk your hands toward your knees and tilt your pelvis forward until you find your edge. Relax your head, neck, and arms, letting gravity do the work. Slightly bend your knees to prevent them from locking up. **Hold.** Inhale and exhale slow, steady breaths through your nose. Slowly reverse out of the pose.

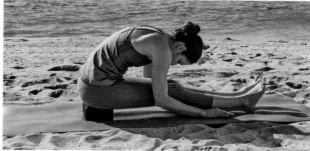

MAKE IT EASIER
In step 1, sit on a block to help your pelvis tilt forward. You can also place a bolster between your chest and legs for more support or you can add a smaller bolster under your knees to keep them bent.

Butterfly

This seated asana provides one of the best stretches for your inner groin while also improving hip flexibility and stretching your lower back. It is also thought to help improve kidney and prostate functions.

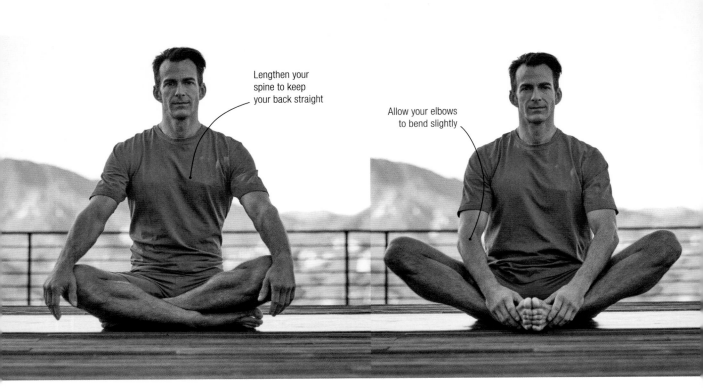

Lengthen your spine to keep your back straight

Allow your elbows to bend slightly

1 Sit on the ground in a comfortable position, crossing your legs and keeping your tailbone on the ground. Put your hands on your knees, and extend the crown of your head upward.

2 Bring the soles of your feet together and use your hands to pull your heels closer to your groin.

BE AWARE If you have sciatica pain, take caution when performing this pose because it can aggravate that condition.

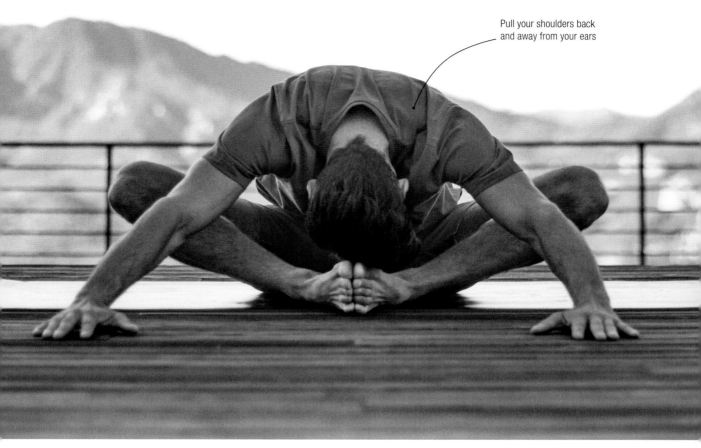

Pull your shoulders back and away from your ears

3 Fold forward from your hips, letting gravity take over until you find your edge. Place your hands out wide in front of you, keeping your palms flat on the ground. Relax your neck and slightly round your spine. **Hold.** Inhale and exhale slow, steady breaths through your nose. Slowly reverse out of the pose.

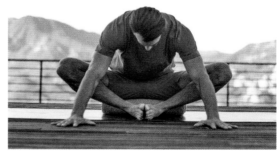

MAKE IT EASIER
In step 3, elevate your hips by sitting on a folded blanket or on a bolster.

Half butterfly

This asana opens your hips through outer hip rotation and stretches deeply into your hamstrings. The forward fold lightly compresses your internal organs, nurturing healthy digestion.

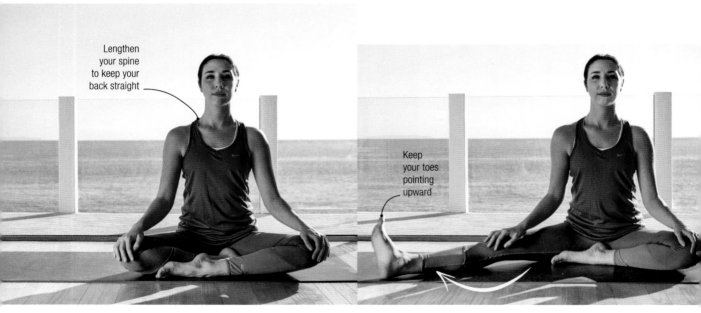

Lengthen your spine to keep your back straight

Keep your toes pointing upward

1 Sit on the ground in a comfortable position, crossing your legs and keeping your tailbone on the ground. Put your hands on your knees and extend the crown of your head upward.

2 Extend your right leg out to the side and bend your left knee to place the sole of your left foot on the inside of your right thigh.

BE AWARE If you have limited hamstring flexibility or have ever suffered a hamstring injury, this pose could cause significant discomfort, so keep a gentle bend in your knees.

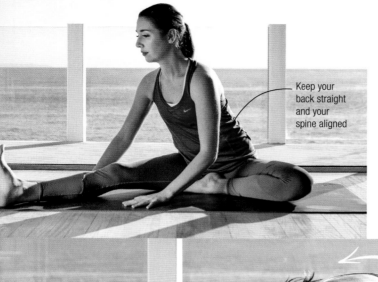

Keep your back straight and your spine aligned

3 Turn your upper body toward your right leg, put your hands on the ground on the sides of your right leg, and slowly walk your hands forward, pressing your left thigh down to keep your tailbone on the ground.

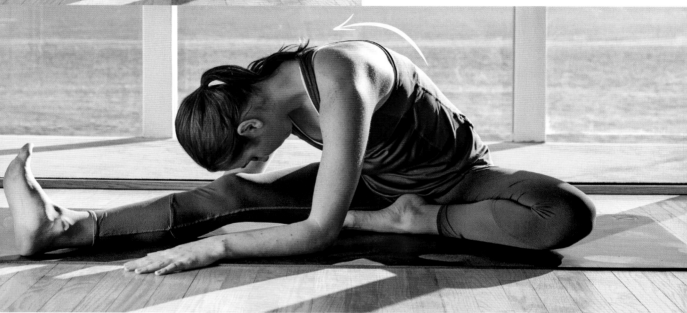

4 Let your upper body relax and your back round as you fold your stomach toward your right thigh until you find your edge. **Hold.** Inhale and exhale slow, steady breaths through your nose. Slowly reverse out of the pose as you return to your starting position, then repeat with the opposite leg.

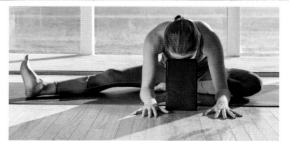

MAKE IT EASIER
In step 4, walk your hands out in front of your hips—rather than turn to the side— and place a block or a bolster under your forehead for support.

Reclined butterfly

This asana is a restorative way to open up your hips and stretch your inner groin as well as improve hip flexibility. Although this pose is mostly passive, it's also intense, so ensure you're in a comfortable position throughout.

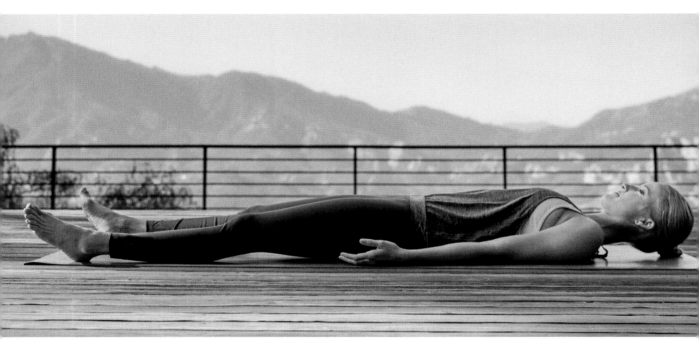

1 Lie on your back, keeping your legs and shoulder blades flat on the ground and relaxing your arms at your sides, with your palms facing up.

BE AWARE This pose requires little effort, but it can put a strain on weakened or injured knees, so place blankets or blocks under your knees to help relieve any discomfort.

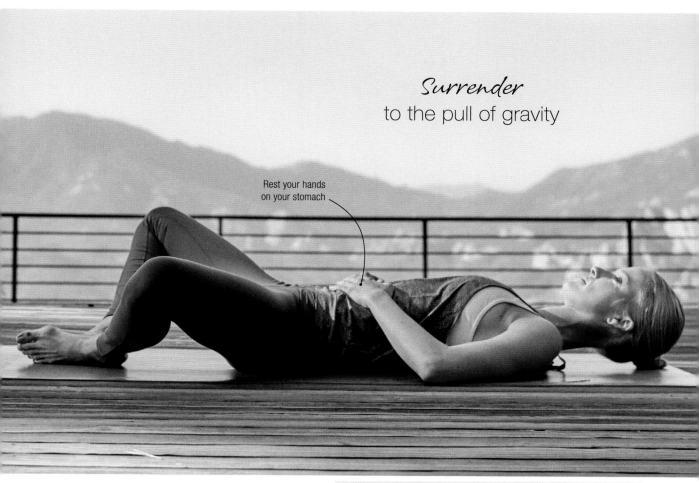

Surrender
to the pull of gravity

Rest your hands
on your stomach

2 Bend your knees so the soles of your feet
touch. Bring your heels closer to your groin,
and relax your legs to let gravity pull them
toward the ground. **Hold.** Inhale and exhale
slow, steady breaths through your nose.
Slowly reverse out of the pose.

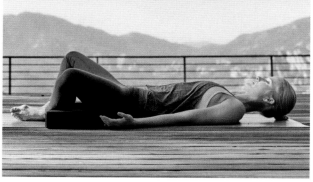

MAKE IT EASIER
In step 2, place a block under each thigh.

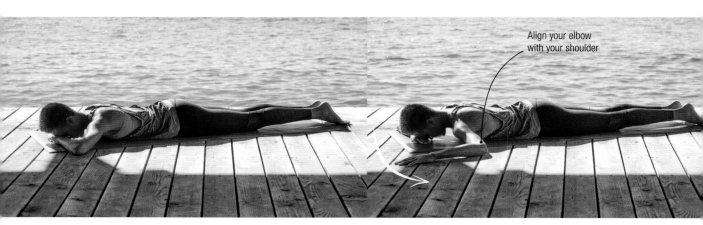

Align your elbow
with your shoulder

1 Lie on your stomach, stack your palms under your forehead, and fully extend your legs behind you.

2 Reach your left arm out to the left, bending your elbow at a 90-degree angle and keeping your left palm flat on the ground.

Lying chest opener

This energizing asana helps counteract the excessive shoulder hunching you do while driving or sitting at a desk.' This pose also improves overall posture and shoulder flexibility while requiring minimal effort.

BE AWARE If you feel a tingling sensation down either arm while performing this asana, carefully reverse your movements to slowly back out of the pose.

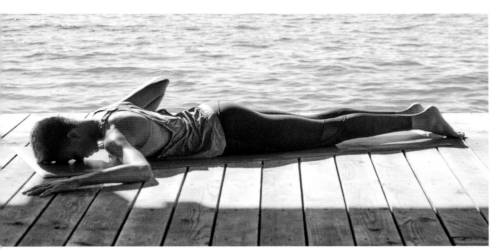

3 Reach your right arm out to your side, bend your right elbow, and place your right hand flat on the ground next to your rib cage.

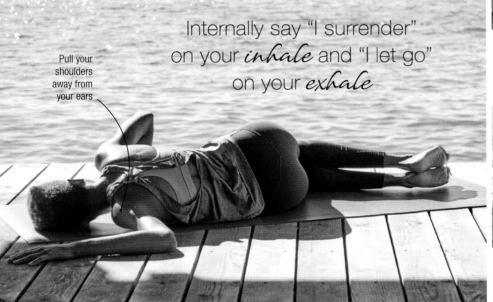

Internally say "I surrender" on your *inhale* and "I let go" on your *exhale*

Pull your shoulders away from your ears

4 Slowly push your right hand into the ground to lift your right side up and roll onto your left ear, shoulder, and hip. Bend your knees slightly and allow your legs to relax, keeping them stacked. **Hold.** Inhale and exhale slow, steady breaths through your nose. Slowly reverse out of the pose as you return to your starting position, then repeat on the opposite side.

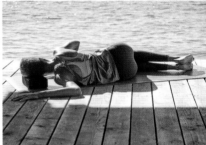

MAKE IT EASIER
In step 4, place a block under your head.

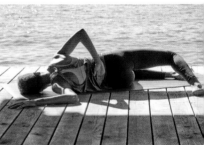

MAKE IT HARDER
In step 4, place the back of the hand of your top arm on your lower back and extend your top leg behind you.

Lying quad stretch

This simple asana opens up your upper legs and can help you prepare for doing backbends. If you're a runner, you'll find this pose quite beneficial to relieve muscular aches and pains in your thighs. You'll also reduce post-workout leg stiffness.

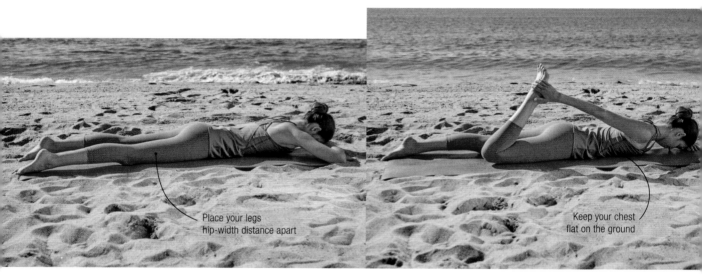

Place your legs hip-width distance apart

Keep your chest flat on the ground

1 Lie on your stomach, stack your hands under your forehead, and fully extend your legs behind you, keeping your toes flat on the ground and your neck and back straight.

2 Bend your right knee to bring your right leg toward your head and reach your right hand behind you to grab the outer side of your right foot.

BE AWARE If you've ever suffered any lower-back injury, use a strap to help make this pose more comfortable.

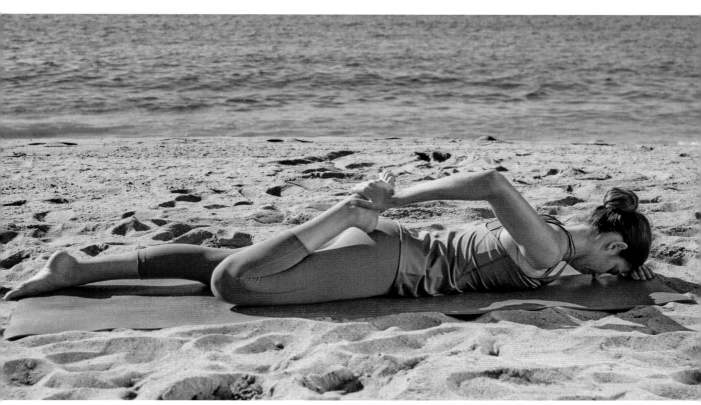

3 Gently pull your right foot toward your glutes and extend your tailbone toward your feet to lengthen the lower back. **Hold.** Inhale and exhale slow, steady breaths through your nose. Slowly reverse out of the pose as you return to your starting position, then repeat with the opposite leg.

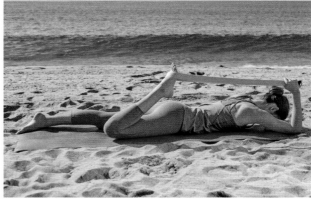

MAKE IT EASIER
In step 3, use a strap around the top of the foot of the bent knee.

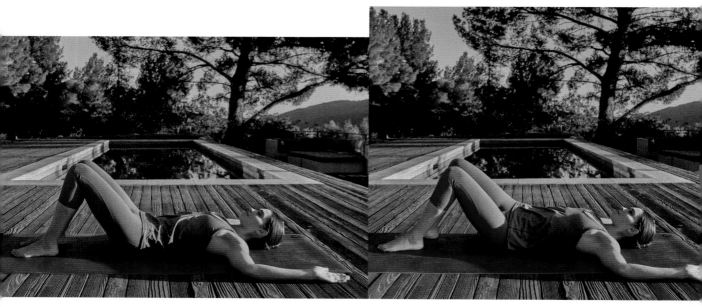

1 Lie on your back and bend your knees, keeping your feet flat on the ground. Place your arms at your sides to create 90-degree angles and face your palms up.

2 Press your feet down into the ground and slide your hips a few inches to your right. Continue to keep your head and shoulder blades flat on the ground.

Lying spinal twist

Supine twists offer a gentle compression of the stomach, which might improve digestion. This particular twist can also stretch your lower back, helping with mobility issues.

BE AWARE Although twists might soothe back pain, you should avoid them if you've suffered any kind of spine injury.

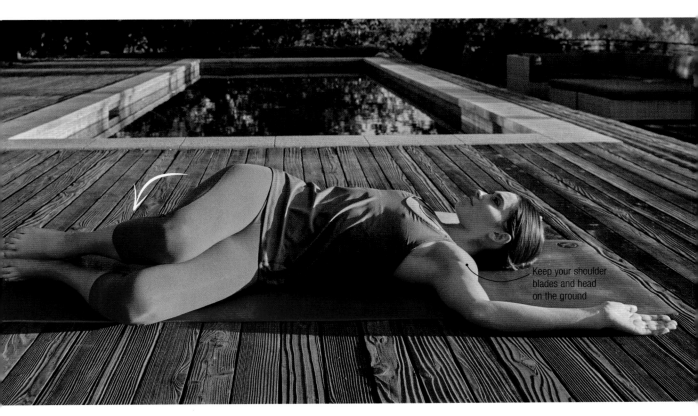

Keep your shoulder
blades and head
on the ground

3 Anchoring your right shoulder blade to the ground, let both legs drop down to your left until your left leg is flat on the ground. **Hold.** Inhale and exhale slow, steady breaths through your nose. Slowly reverse out of the pose as you return to your starting position, then repeat on the opposite side.

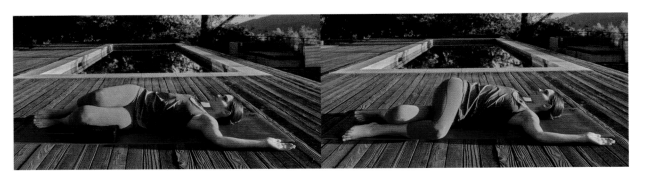

MAKE IT EASIER
In step 3, place a block under your knees.

MAKE IT HARDER
In step 3, cross your top thigh over your bottom thigh—but don't alter the position of your shoulders.

Saddle

This asana opens up the front of your thighs and stretches your ankle and knee joints through inner hip rotation. This pose will also stretch your quadriceps, hip flexors, and shoulders for a full-body experience.

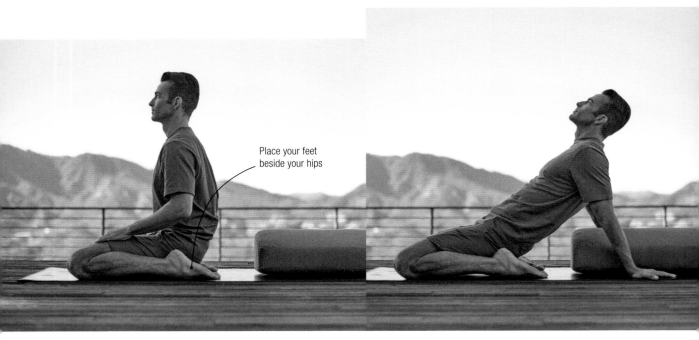

Place your feet beside your hips

1 Place a bolster behind you. Sit in a kneeling position, put your legs outside your hips, and keep your tailbone on the ground. Keep the tops of your feet flat on the ground and point your toes straight back. Lengthen your spine and rest your palms on your thighs.

2 Extend your arms behind you and walk your hands toward the bolster. Extend your tailbone toward your heels to lengthen your lower back and keep your legs flat on the ground. Keep your back and neck straight as you begin to lower yourself onto the bolster behind you.

BE AWARE If you feel pain in your knees and ankles or have suffered knee or ankle injuries, use a blanket or a bolster for support.

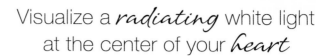

Visualize a *radiating* white light
at the center of your *heart*

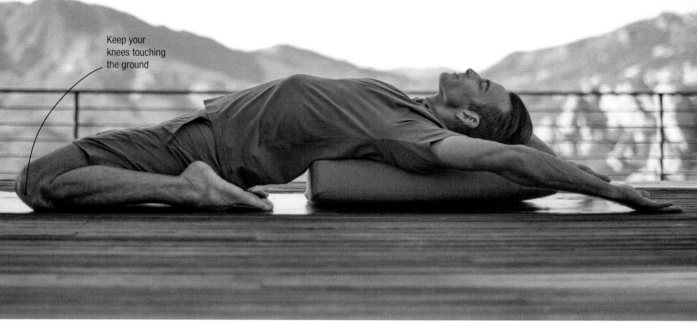

Keep your
knees touching
the ground

3 Lower all the way down to the bolster (or go all the way to the ground) and extend your arms over your head to stretch your chest and shoulders. **Hold.** Inhale and exhale slow, steady breaths through your nose. Slowly reverse out of the pose.

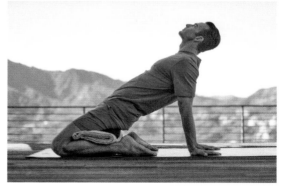

MAKE IT EASIER
In step 3, put a blanket and a block behind your thighs and on top of the back of your calves to keep your hips elevated. Walk your hands behind you and hold yourself up.

Archer arms

This asana encourages deep breathing by opening up your chest and improving flexibility in your shoulders. You'll also feel your upper arms and upper back stretch and strengthen.

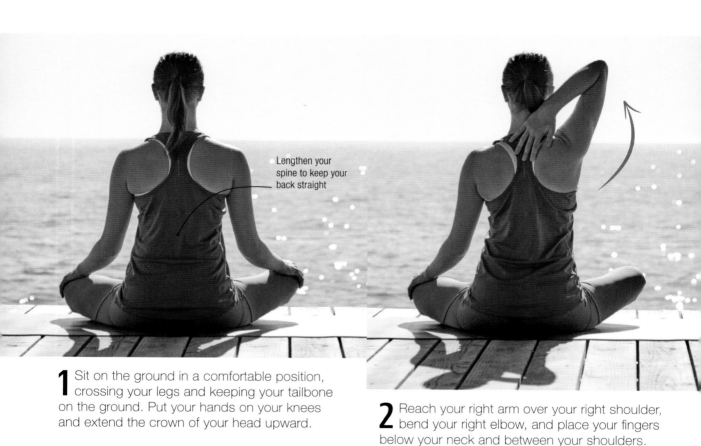

Lengthen your spine to keep your back straight

1 Sit on the ground in a comfortable position, crossing your legs and keeping your tailbone on the ground. Put your hands on your knees and extend the crown of your head upward.

2 Reach your right arm over your right shoulder, bend your right elbow, and place your fingers below your neck and between your shoulders.

BE AWARE If you've had any kind of shoulder injury, this pose might aggravate that injury. You might find that using a strap will help alleviate some discomfort.

Feel your rib cage *expand* from front to back and side to side as you *breathe in and out* through your nose

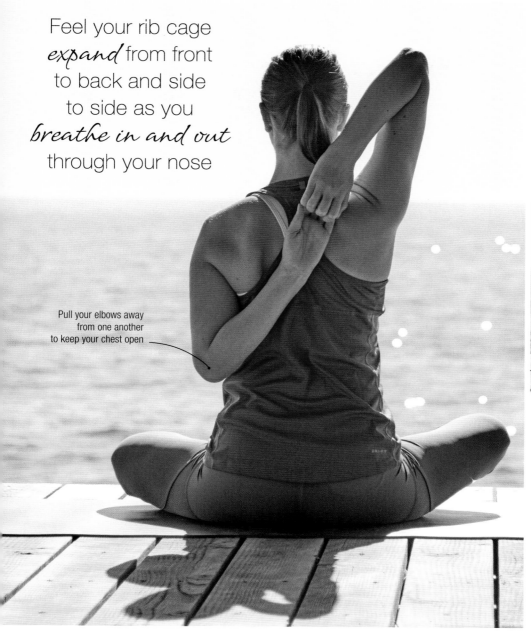

Pull your elbows away from one another to keep your chest open

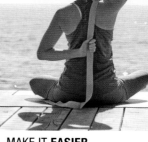

MAKE IT EASIER
In step 3, hold a strap in both hands.

3 Reach your left arm behind your back, bend your left elbow, and reach your left hand up to your right hand to interlace your fingers. **Hold.** Inhale and exhale slow, steady breaths through your nose. Slowly reverse out of the pose as you return to your starting position, then switch the arm positions and repeat.

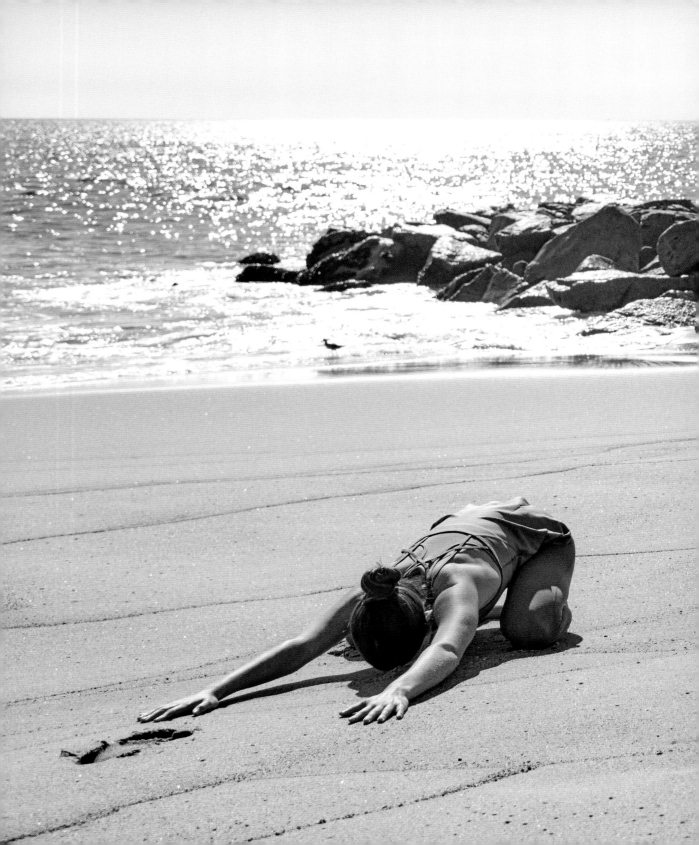

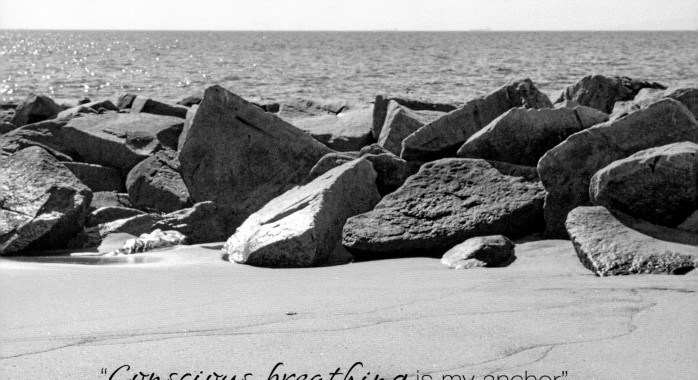

"*Conscious breathing* is my anchor"

Thich Nhat Hanh

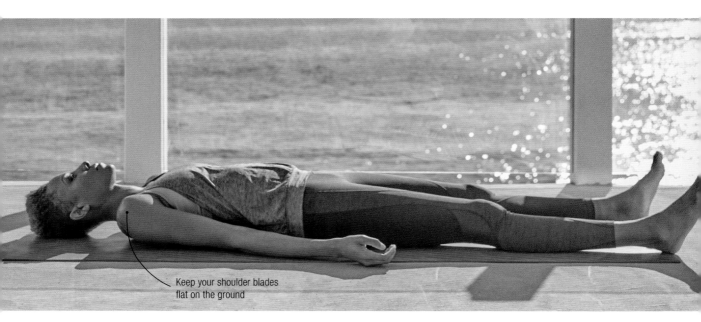

Keep your shoulder blades
flat on the ground

1 Lie on your back and extend your legs straight
out in front of you, keeping your feet hip-width
distance apart.

Knee to chest

This gentle hip-opening asana lightly stretches your lower back
and compresses your stomach to encourage healthy digestion.
You can practice this pose as a morning warmup or before bed.

BE AWARE If you've ever suffered any kind of spinal or knee injury,
use caution while performing this asana.

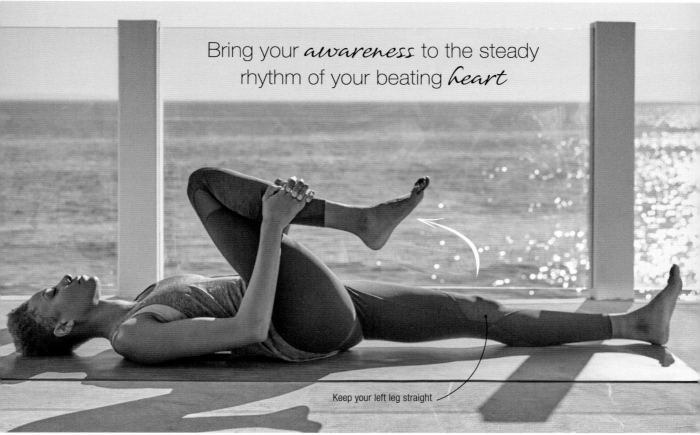

Bring your *awareness* to the steady
rhythm of your beating *heart*

Keep your left leg straight

2 Wrap your hands around your right shin
and pull your right knee into your chest.
Press down through your left heel to keep
your left leg extended and soften your
shoulders, keeping them in contact with
the ground. **Hold.** Inhale and exhale slow,
steady breaths through your nose. Slowly
reverse out of the pose as you return to
your starting position, then repeat with the
opposite leg.

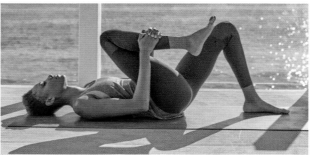

MAKE IT EASIER
In step 2, bend your left knee and keep your left
foot flat on the ground as you pull your right knee
toward your stomach.

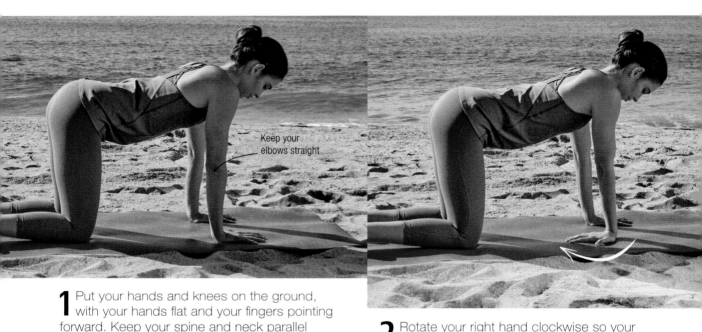

Keep your
elbows straight

1 Put your hands and knees on the ground,
with your hands flat and your fingers pointing
forward. Keep your spine and neck parallel
to the ground and your eyes looking down.

2 Rotate your right hand clockwise so your
fingertips point toward your right knee.
Spread your fingers wide to keep your weight
evenly distributed throughout your hands.

Wrist flexor stretch

This simple stretch will free up your wrists and forearms
to soothe aching joints, especially if you suffer from
carpal tunnel syndrome.

BE AWARE If you've ever suffered any kind of wrist injury, you might want
to avoid this stretch. Go slowly—and stop if you experience any pain.

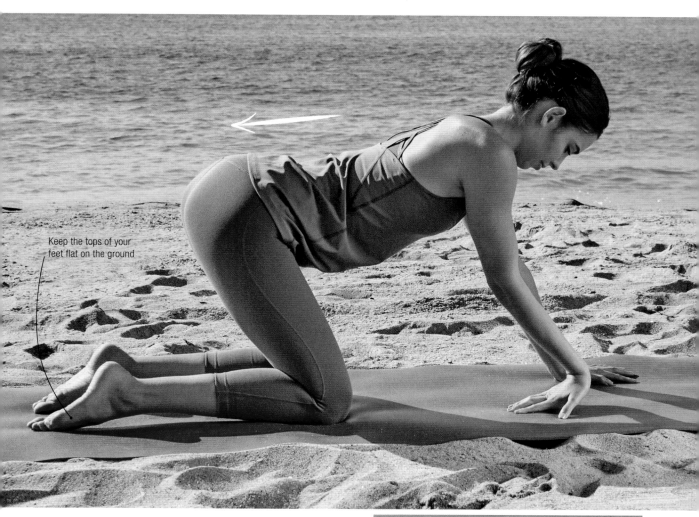

Keep the tops of your feet flat on the ground

3 Slowly shift your weight back toward your heels and lift your right palm off the ground, keeping your fingertips and your left hand flat on the ground. **Hold.** Inhale and exhale slow, steady breaths through your nose. Slowly reverse out of the pose as you return to your starting position, then repeat with the opposite hand.

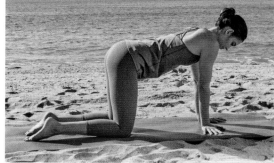

MAKE IT EASIER
In step 2, rotate your fingers toward the outer sides of the mat.

Wrist extensor stretch

This asana will help improve your wrist mobility and deeply stretch your forearms. This pose is especially beneficial if you suffer from tennis elbow.

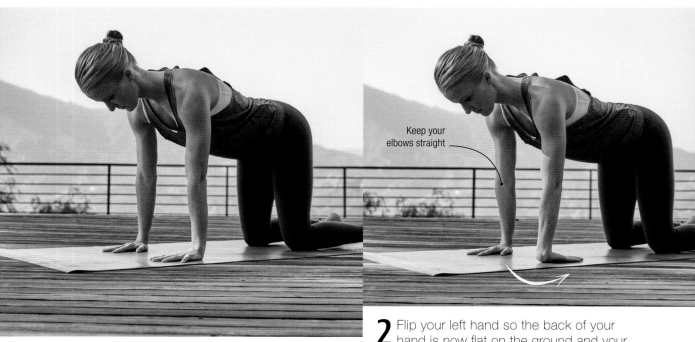

Keep your elbows straight

1 Put your hands and knees on the ground, with your hands flat and your fingers pointing forward. Keep your spine and neck parallel to the ground and your eyes looking down.

2 Flip your left hand so the back of your hand is now flat on the ground and your fingertips point toward your left knee. Spread your fingers wide and keep your weight evenly distributed throughout your hands.

BE AWARE If you've ever suffered any kind of wrist injury, you might want to avoid this stretch. Go slowly—and stop if you experience any pain.

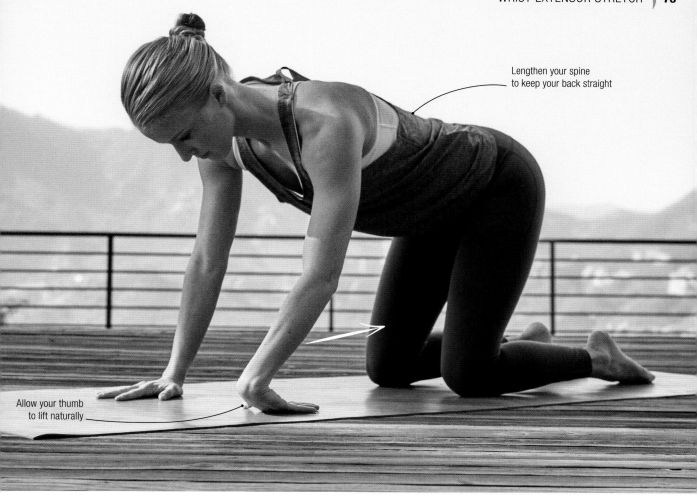

Lengthen your spine
to keep your back straight

Allow your thumb
to lift naturally

3 Slowly shift your weight back toward your heels
and lift the back of your left hand off the ground
while keeping your knuckles and your right hand
flat on the ground. **Hold.** Inhale and exhale slow,
steady breaths through your nose. Slowly reverse
out of the pose as you return to your starting
position, then repeat with the opposite hand.

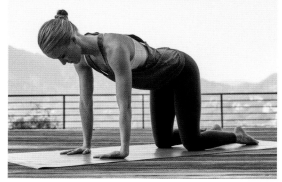

MAKE IT EASIER
In step 2, rotate your fingers toward the
center of the mat after flipping your hand.

Sphinx

This heart-opening asana will help you learn to breathe deeply into your chest and upper back while providing a backbend that might help reduce lower-back pain and improve spine flexibility.

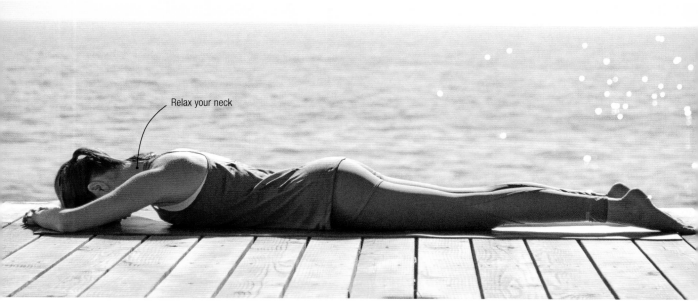

Relax your neck

1 Lie on your stomach, bending your elbows at 90-degree angles and stacking your hands in front of your head. Keep your hands and forearms flat on the ground. Rest your forehead on the ground and fully extend your legs behind you.

BE AWARE If you've ever suffered any kind of back injury, use caution when doing backbends. Go slowly—and stop if you experience any pain.

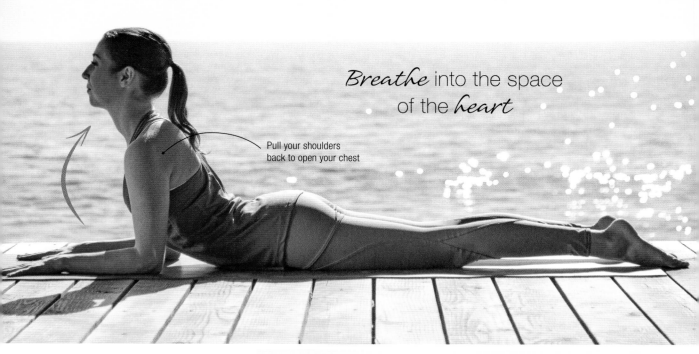

Breathe into the space
of the *heart*

Pull your shoulders
back to open your chest

2 Press your forearms into the
ground and slide your hands
back to lift up your head and
chest. Align your elbows with
your shoulders and spread your
fingers wide. Extend your tailbone
toward your heels and pull your
chest forward, relaxing your upper
body as much as possible. **Hold.**
Inhale and exhale slow, steady
breaths through your nose.
Slowly reverse out of the pose.

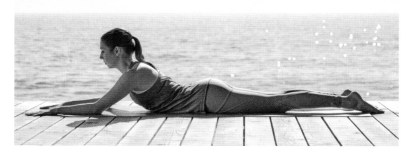

MAKE IT EASIER
In step 2, slide your arms farther forward.

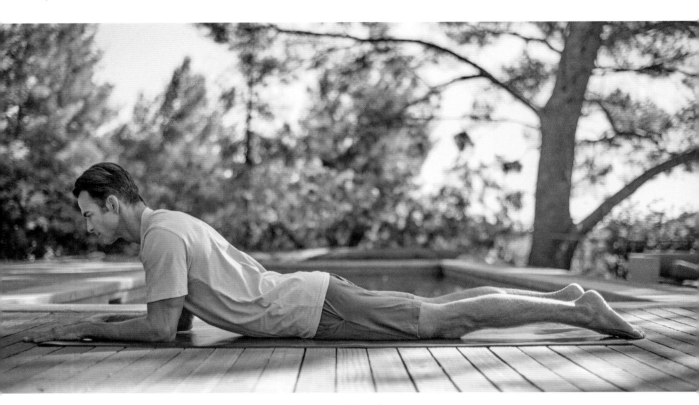

1 Lie on your stomach, bending your elbows and keeping your hands and forearms flat on the ground in front of you. Press your forearms into the ground to lift your chest and head, and fully extend your legs behind you.

Seal

This asana is similar to the Sphinx pose, but it provides a much deeper backbend and might help with digestion. This is a great pose to do if you spend long hours sitting in a chair because it reinforces the natural curve of your lower back.

BE AWARE If you experience pain in your lower back or sacrum while performing this pose, perform the Sphinx pose (page 74) instead.

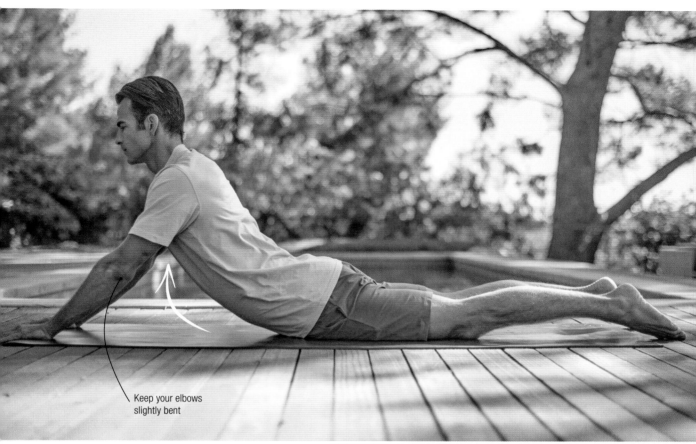

Keep your elbows
slightly bent

2 Press your palms into the ground to lift your arms and chest off the ground, broadening your chest and pulling your shoulders back. **Hold.** Inhale and exhale slow, steady breaths through your nose. Slowly reverse out of the pose.

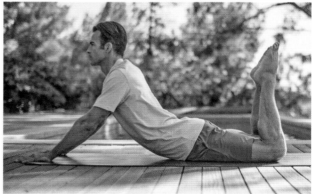

MAKE IT EASIER
In step 2, bend both knees as if you're going to touch your toes to your head, but keep your hips firmly planted on the ground.

Side seal

This asana is a variation of the classic Seal pose and helps to open up the side body in a restorative way. Side bends are a great way to boost your energy, and they also support healthy digestion as well as improve your lateral spine flexibility.

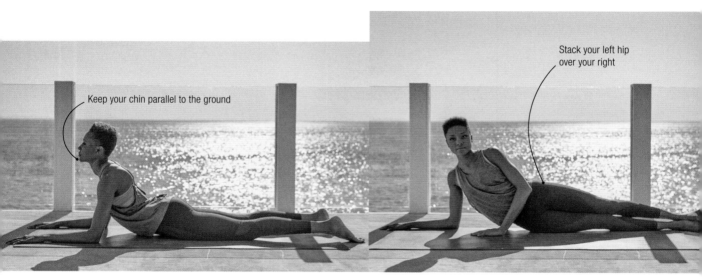

Keep your chin parallel to the ground

Stack your left hip over your right

1 Lie on your stomach and fully extend your legs behind you. Bend your elbows and keep your hands and forearms flat on the ground in front of you. Press your forearms into the ground to lift your chest and head off the ground.

2 Push on the ground with your left hand to roll onto your right hip and right forearm, keeping your legs extended and aligning your left leg on top of your right. Pull your shoulder blades back and lift your chest, placing your left hand flat on the ground in front of you for stability.

BE AWARE You can place a folded blanket under your hips if you feel discomfort in that area while holding the pose.

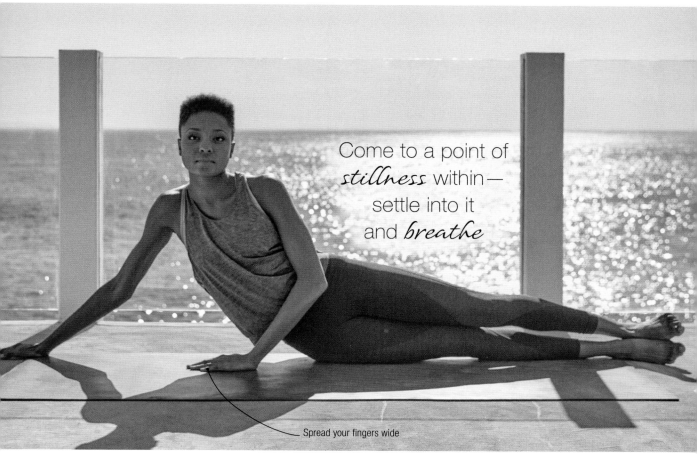

Come to a point of stillness *within— settle into it and* breathe

Spread your fingers wide

3 Press your right hand into the ground to straighten your right arm and extend your tailbone toward your heels. Pull the crown of your head upward. **Hold.** Inhale and exhale slow, steady breaths through your nose. Slowly reverse out of the pose as you return to your starting position, then repeat on the opposite side.

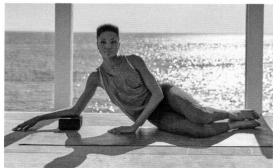

MAKE IT EASIER
In step 2, bend your knees and place a block under the elbow of the extended arm for more support.

Banana

This beginner-friendly asana will give you a deep side stretch from your armpits to your legs, including your IT band and obliques areas. Performing this in the morning can invigorate you for your entire day.

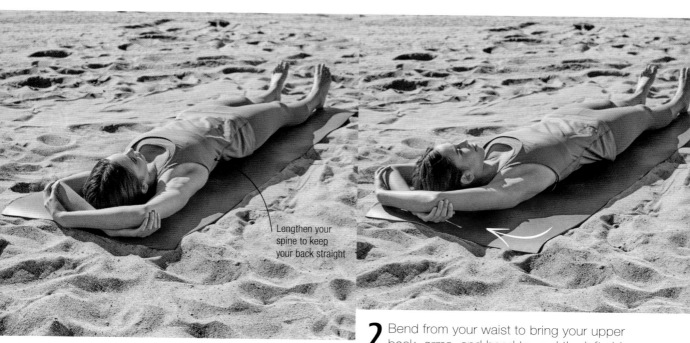

Lengthen your spine to keep your back straight

1 Lie on your back, extending your legs straight out in front of you. Reaching your arms over your head, grab your opposite elbows with your hands.

2 Bend from your waist to bring your upper back, arms, and head toward the left side of the mat, keeping your legs straight and your hips on the ground.

BE AWARE If you feel any discomfort in your arms or shoulders, keep your arms by your sides instead.

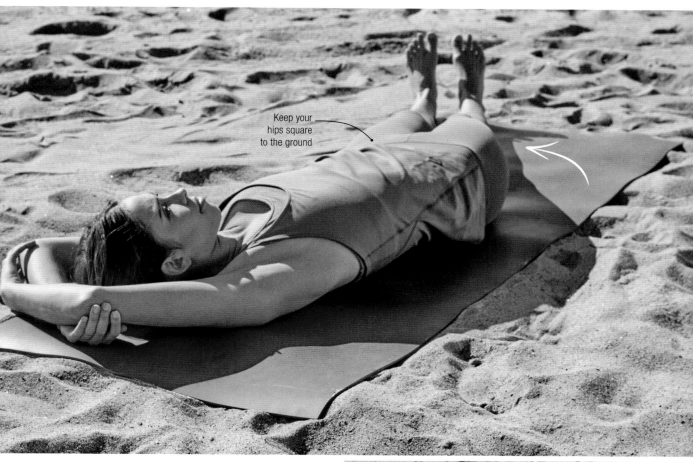

Keep your hips square to the ground

3 Complete the side bend by pressing your hips into the mat and walking your feet to the left until you form a banana shape with your body. **Hold.** Inhale and exhale slow, steady breaths through your nose. Slowly reverse out of the pose as you return to your starting position, then repeat on the opposite side.

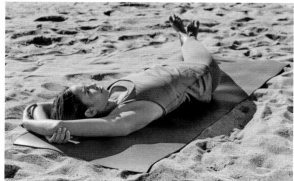

MAKE IT HARDER
In step 3, deepen the stretch in your IT band by crossing your right ankle over your left ankle without lifting your right hip off the ground.

Straddle

This forward fold opens up your inner legs to improve lower-body flexibility while decompressing your spine. This is also a great pose to do after a strong workout.

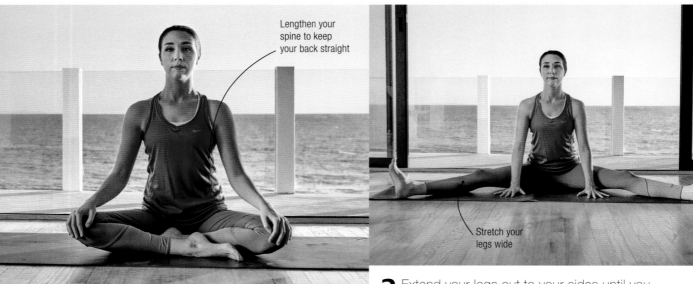

Lengthen your spine to keep your back straight

Stretch your legs wide

1 Sit on the ground in a comfortable position, crossing your legs and keeping your tailbone on the ground. Put your hands on your knees and extend the crown of your head upward.

2 Extend your legs out to your sides until you find your edge. Put your hands flat on the ground in front of you, with your fingers pointing forward, and keep your toes pointing straight up.

BE AWARE Although folding forward could aggravate lower-back injuries or sciatica, you can sit on a block or folded blankets to elevate your hips or you can avoid folding forward altogether.

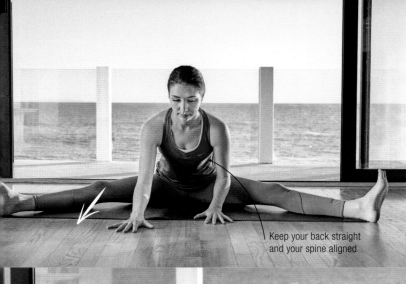

3 Tilt your pelvis forward to initiate the forward fold and walk your hands out in front of you for support.

Keep your back straight and your spine aligned

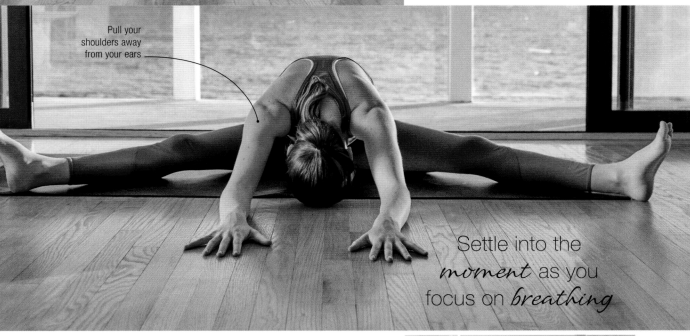

Pull your shoulders away from your ears

Settle into the *moment* as you focus on *breathing*

4 Once you find your edge, allow your spine to round slightly. Allow gravity to pull you closer to the ground. **Hold.** Inhale and exhale slow, steady breaths through your nose. Slowly reverse out of the pose.

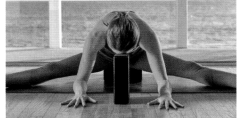

MAKE IT EASIER
In step 3, prop your hips up on a block to help you tilt your pelvis forward and place a block on its short side under your forehead for support.

Dangling

This asana is the only one in this book you can do standing up, but it's a great way to lengthen your spine and stretch your hamstrings. Perform this forward fold to restore energy levels after a long day.

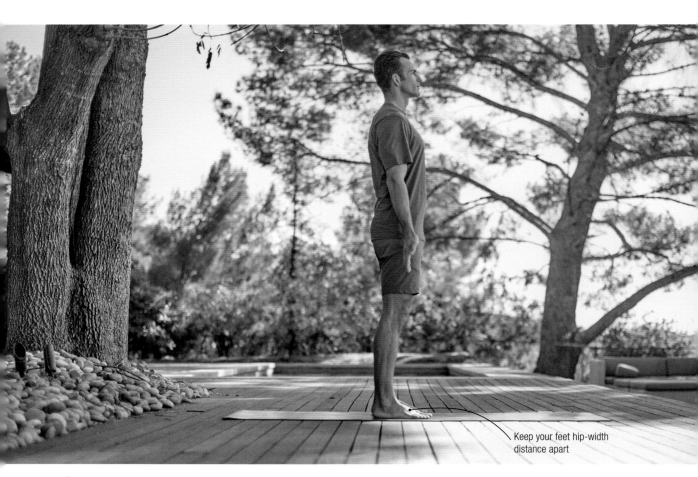

Keep your feet hip-width distance apart

1 Stand tall, lengthening your spine, gently bending your knees, and relaxing your arms at your sides, with your palms facing forward.

BE AWARE If you've suffered any kind of lower-back injury, you can bend your knees more or you might want to avoid this pose if you experience any pain.

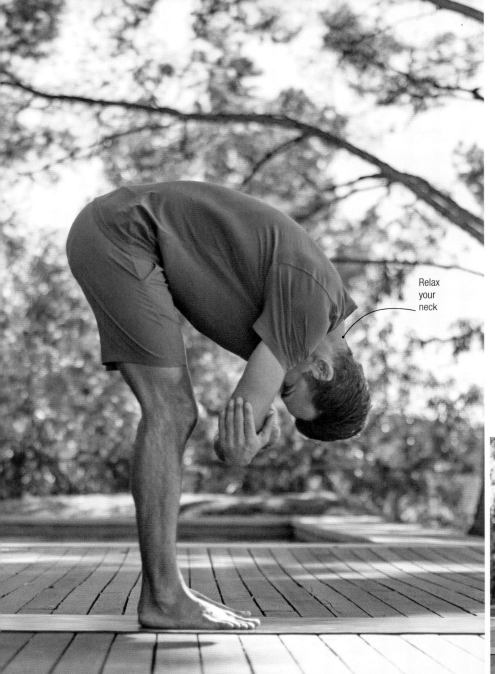

Imagine *stress pouring out* from the top of your head with every exhale

Relax your neck

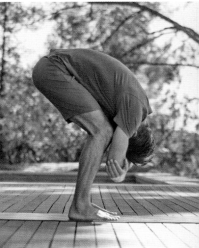

MAKE IT EASIER
In step 2, bend your knees even more to better support yourself during the fold.

2 Fold forward at your hips, maintaining the gentle bend in your knees, and wrap your hands around the opposite elbows. Keep your weight evenly distributed throughout your feet, but allow gravity to take over. **Hold.** Inhale and exhale slow, steady breaths through your nose. Slowly reverse out of the pose.

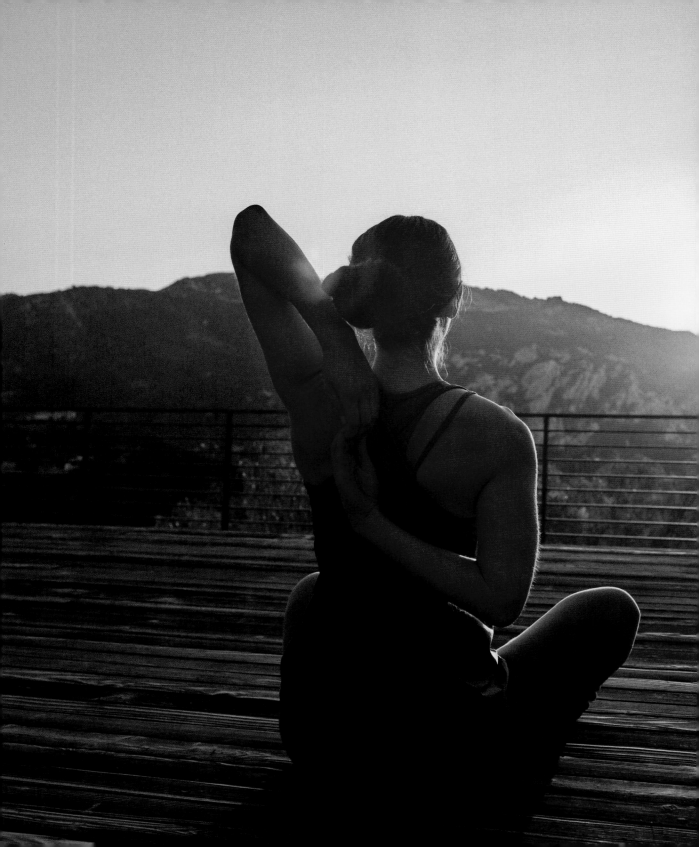

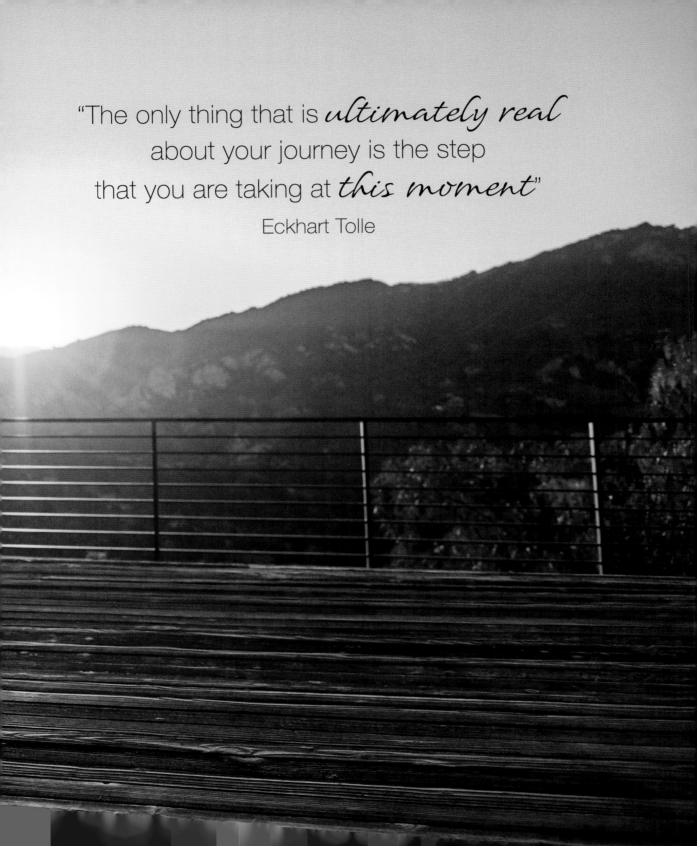

Snail

This intense asana provides the benefits of a forward fold combined with an inversion. It's a powerful way to stretch the back of your body—from the crown of your head, down your spine, and into your hamstrings.

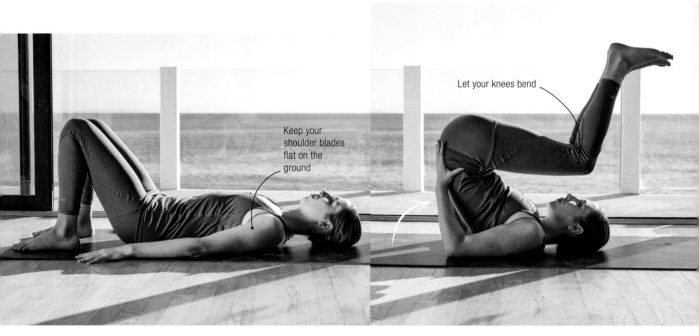

Keep your shoulder blades flat on the ground

Let your knees bend

1 Lie on your back and bend your knees, with your feet flat on the ground. Relax your arms at your sides and keep your hands flat on the ground.

2 Lift your hips and feet up so your knees move toward your head and place your hands behind your lower back. Let your spine and legs round to find your balance.

BE AWARE If you've ever suffered any kind of neck injury or if you suffer from glaucoma, you should avoid this pose because it could aggravate these conditions.

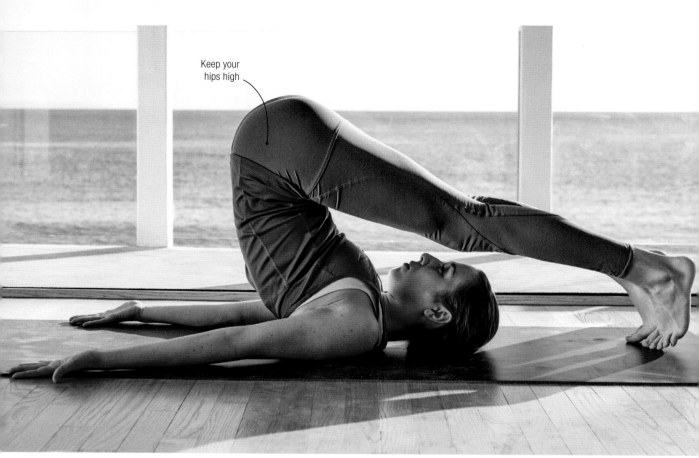

Keep your
hips high

3 Straighten your legs back over your head
so your toes touch the ground behind you.
Keep your hips elevated and straighten your
arms out in front of you, with your palms facing
up for stability. **Hold.** Inhale and exhale slow,
steady breaths through your nose. Slowly
reverse out of the pose.

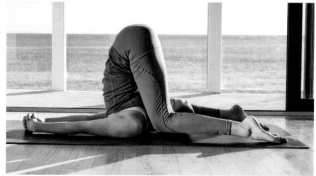

MAKE IT HARDER
In step 3, bend your knees and rest them beside
your ears, keeping your knees and the tops of
your feet flat on the ground. Interlace your fingers,
keeping your arms straight out in front of you and
your elbows unbent.

Baby dragon

This asana does wonders for anyone who spends many hours sitting in a chair, and it might also prove therapeutic for sciatica pain. It stretches deeply into the front of your hips and creates length in your lower back.

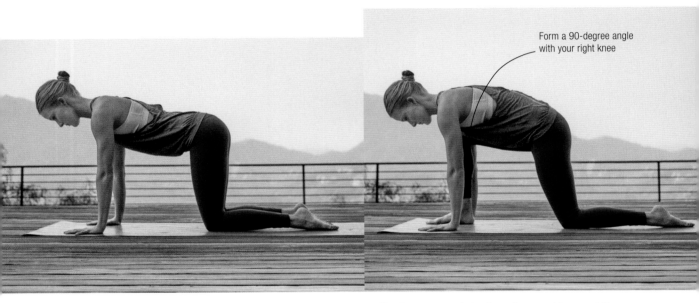

Form a 90-degree angle with your right knee

1 Put your hands and knees on the ground, with your hands flat and your fingers pointing forward. Keep your spine and neck parallel to the ground and your eyes looking down.

2 Step your right foot forward toward the top corner of your mat and positioned to the inside of your right hand, aligning your right knee directly over your right ankle.

BE AWARE If you have knee sensitivities or have ever suffered any kind of knee injury, you might find this uncomfortable and should perform the Knee to chest (page 84) instead.

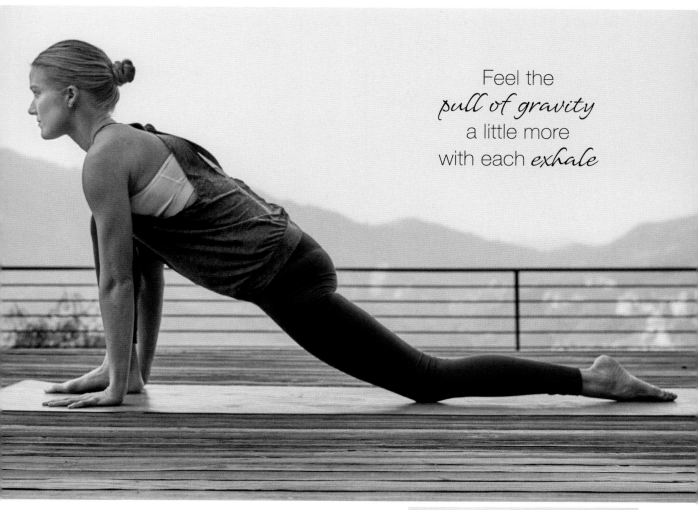

Feel the
pull of gravity
a little more
with each *exhale*

3 Extend your left leg behind you, allowing your hips to drop down. Keep your left knee on the ground and your arms straight and lift your head to look forward. Press down on your right big toe to keep your right foot flat on the ground and let gravity pull your hips down. **Hold.** Inhale and exhale slow, steady breaths through your nose. Slowly reverse out of the pose as you return to your starting position, then repeat with the opposite leg.

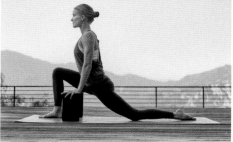

MAKE IT EASIER
In step 3, place a block under each hand to keep your chest elevated.

Twisted dragon

This asana helps you go even deeper into your legs by targeting your quadriceps. It also opens up your upper body and might provide some relief for lower-back pain.

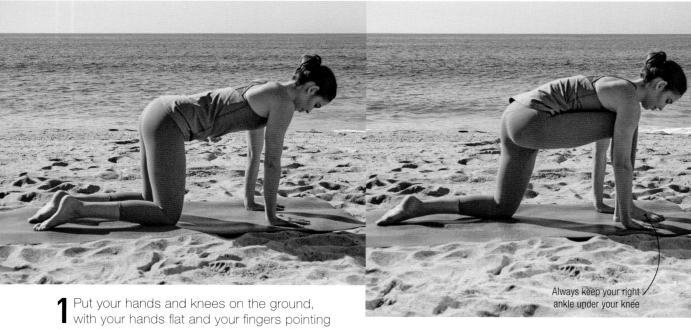

Always keep your right ankle under your knee

1 Put your hands and knees on the ground, with your hands flat and your fingers pointing forward. Keep your spine and neck parallel to the ground and your eyes looking down.

2 Step your right foot forward toward the top corner of your mat and positioned to the inside of your right hand, aligning your right knee directly over your right ankle.

BE AWARE If you have knee sensitivities or have suffered any kind of knee injury, you might find this pose uncomfortable and should perform the Lying quad stretch (page 58) instead.

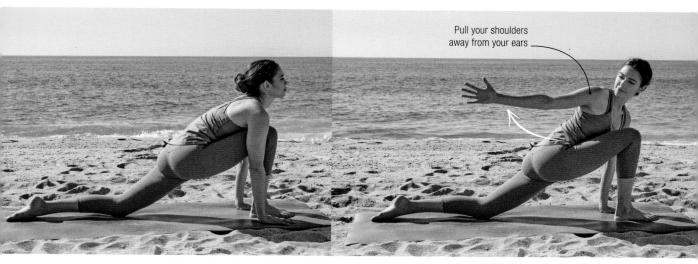

Pull your shoulders
away from your ears

3 Extend your left leg behind you, allowing your hips to drop down. Keep your left knee on the ground.

4 Keep your left palm anchored to the ground and extend your right arm toward the back of your mat, twisting your upper body to the right.

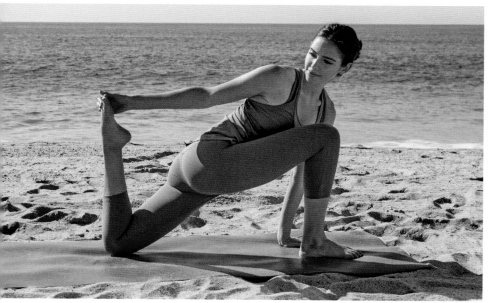

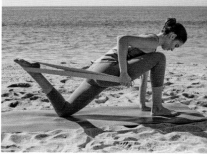

MAKE IT EASIER
In step 5, use a strap around the top of your back foot.

5 Bend your left knee and grab the top of your left foot with your right hand, pulling your left heel closer to your glutes. Soften your shoulders and allow gravity to pull your hips down. **Hold.** Inhale and exhale slow, steady breaths through your nose. Slowly reverse out of the pose as you return to your starting position, then repeat with the opposite leg.

Dragon flying low

This asana goes deeper than the Baby dragon pose by applying more body weight to the hips. It's an intense hip-opening pose that deeply stretches your inner groin and hip flexors to increase mobility in your lower body.

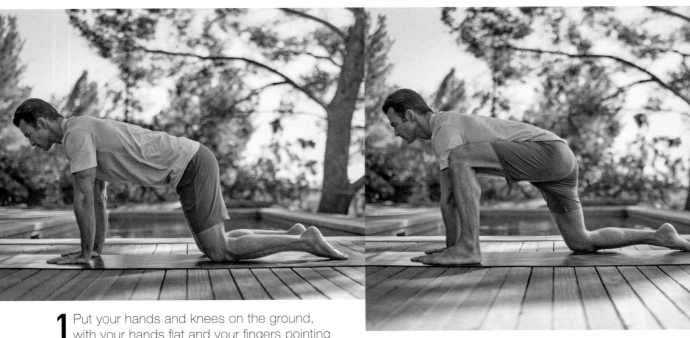

1 Put your hands and knees on the ground, with your hands flat and your fingers pointing forward. Keep your spine and neck parallel to the ground and your eyes looking down.

2 Step your left foot forward toward the top corner of your mat and positioned to the outside of your left hand, aligning your left knee directly over your left ankle.

BE AWARE If you have knee sensitivities or have ever suffered any kind of knee injury, you can place folded blankets under your knees.

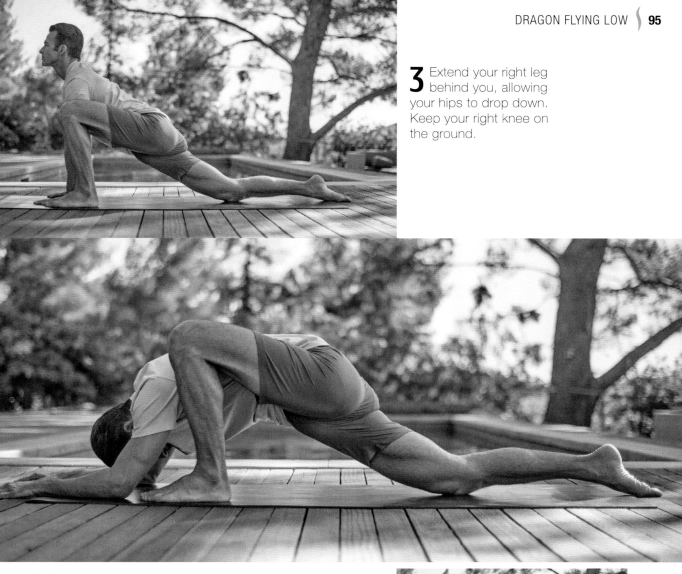

3 Extend your right leg behind you, allowing your hips to drop down. Keep your right knee on the ground.

4 Slide your hands forward to put your forearms flat on the ground. Allow your neck to relax so your head hangs heavy. Press down on your left big toe to keep your left foot flat on the ground and let gravity pull your hips down. **Hold.** Inhale and exhale slow, steady breaths through your nose. Slowly reverse out of the pose as you return to your starting position, then repeat with the opposite leg.

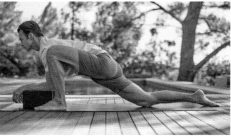

MAKE IT EASIER
In step 4, place your forearms on two blocks or a bolster for support.

Winged dragon

This asana focuses on the outer rotation of your front hip to target the outer portion of your hip socket. It thus provides a very deep stretch for increased flexibility.

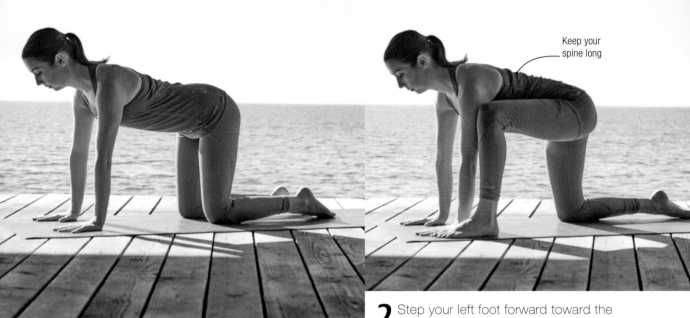

Keep your spine long

1 Put your hands and knees on the ground, with your hands flat and your fingers pointing forward. Keep your spine and neck parallel to the ground and your eyes looking down.

2 Step your left foot forward toward the top corner of your mat and positioned to the outside of your left hand, aligning your left knee directly over your left ankle.

BE AWARE If you have knee, ankle, or hip sensitivities or have ever suffered any kind of injury in these areas, perform the Sleeping swan (page 116) instead.

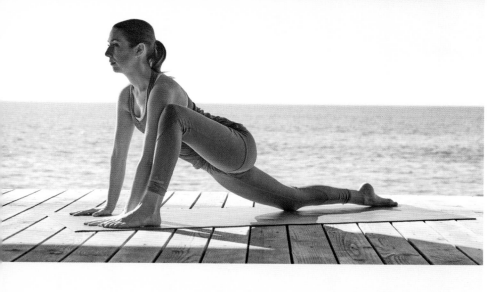

3 Extend your right leg behind you, allowing your hips to drop down. Keep your right knee on the ground as you lift your head to look forward.

Internally repeat
"I am present"
with every exhale

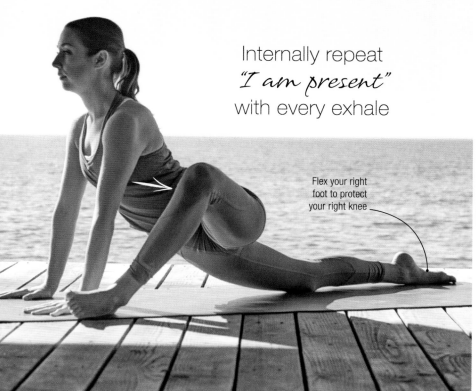

Flex your right foot to protect your right knee

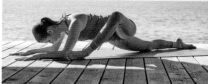

MAKE IT HARDER
In step 4, go deeper into your hip socket by sliding your hands forward so your forearms are flat on the ground. Let your eyes look down. You can place a block under your forehead or you can let your head hang heavy by relaxing your neck.

4 Externally rotate the front of your left hip by rolling your left foot onto its outer side and let gravity pull your left leg down. **Hold.** Inhale and exhale slow, steady breaths through your nose. Slowly reverse out of the pose as you return to your starting position, then repeat with the opposite leg.

Supported bridge

This simple asana offers an easy inversion—perfect for yin yoga beginners. It's a great pose to do if you suffer from lower-back discomfort or simply need to unwind after a long day. You'll need a block for this pose.

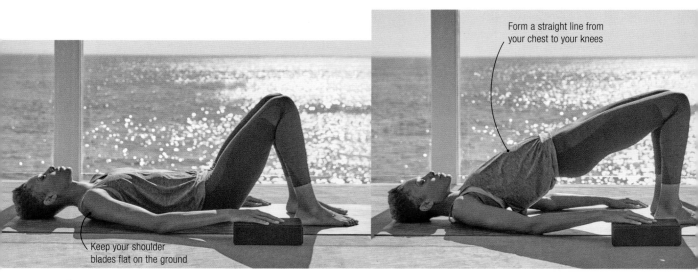

Form a straight line from your chest to your knees

Keep your shoulder blades flat on the ground

1 Lie on your back and bend your knees, keeping your feet flat on the ground. Relax your arms at your sides, with your left hand flat on the ground and a block under your right hand.

2 Press your feet into the ground to lift your hips off the ground and use your core to help push through your feet.

BE AWARE If you have spine issues or have ever suffered any kind of spine injury, use caution when doing backbends.

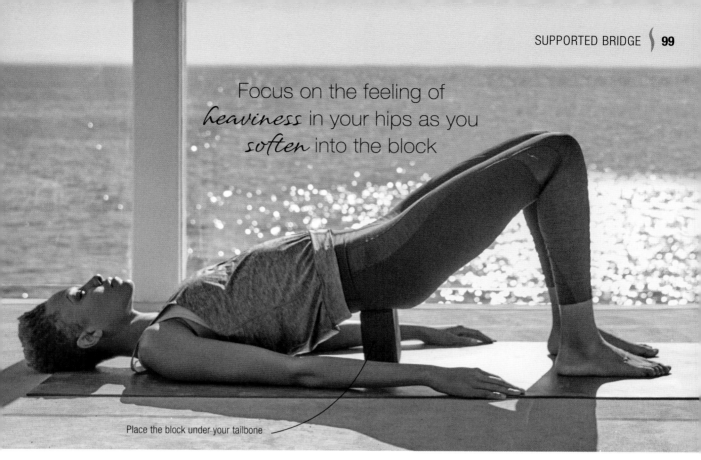

Focus on the feeling of
heaviness in your hips as you
soften into the block

Place the block under your tailbone

3 Position the block on its long side and place it directly under your hips. Rest your hips on the block and relax your arms by your sides. Keep your knees bent and your feet flat on the ground. **Hold.** Inhale and exhale slow, steady breaths through your nose. Slowly reverse out of the pose.

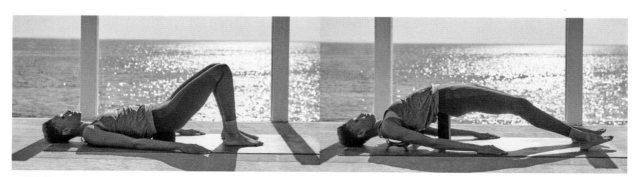

MAKE IT EASIER
In step 3, position your block flat on the ground under your hips.

MAKE IT HARDER
In step 3, position your block on the short side and straighten your legs out in front of you to stretch your hip flexors.

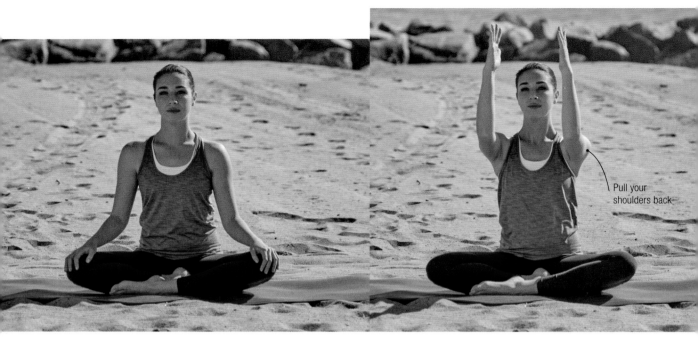

Pull your
shoulders back

1 Sit in a comfortable position, putting your hands on your knees. Keep your tailbone on the ground, cross your legs, and extend the crown of your head upward.

2 Reach your arms up in front of you and bend your elbows at 90-degree angles, aligning them with your shoulders. Face your palms toward each other.

Eagle arms

This upper-body asana broadens the space between your shoulder blades to enable deeper breathing. If you have tight shoulders from working at a desk or suffer from tension-induced headaches, you'll benefit greatly from this pose.

BE AWARE If you've ever suffered any kind of rotator cuff injury, you should avoid this pose, especially if it causes you any pain.

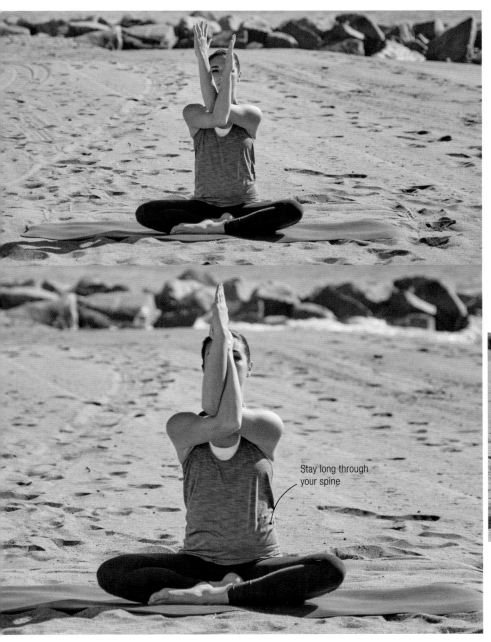

3 Wrap your right arm under your left elbow and bring your right arm up until your forearms are parallel with your body.

Stay long through your spine

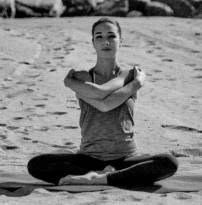

MAKE IT EASIER
In step 3, reach your hands to your opposite shoulders as if giving yourself a big hug. In step 4, hold this position.

4 Wrap your right wrist counterclockwise around your left wrist and place your palms together. Pull your shoulders down from your ears and push your elbows forward. **Hold.** Inhale and exhale slow, steady breaths through your nose. Slowly reverse out of the pose as you return to your starting position, then switch the arm positions and repeat.

Happy baby

This classic asana is a soothing way to target the muscles around your lower back while deeply opening up your hips and inner groin. It's an excellent pose to do first thing in the morning for an all-around stretch.

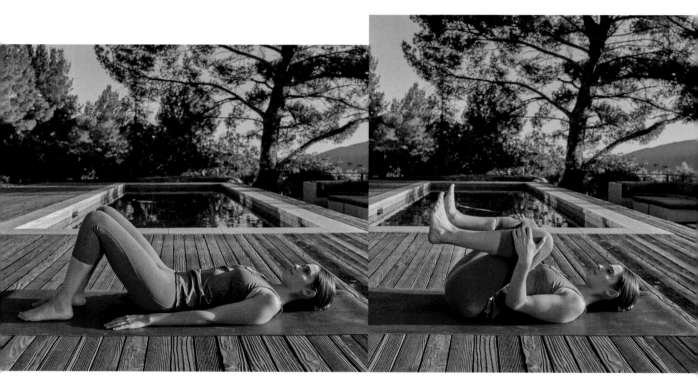

1 Lie on your back and bend your knees, with your feet flat on the ground. Relax your arms at your sides and keep your hands flat on the ground.

2 Bring your knees toward your chest and wrap your hands below your knees, opening them wide to bring them toward your shoulders and armpits. Press your tailbone into the ground to keep your spine level.

BE AWARE If you have neck sensitivities or have ever suffered any kind of neck injury, you can place a folded blanket or a block under your head for extra support.

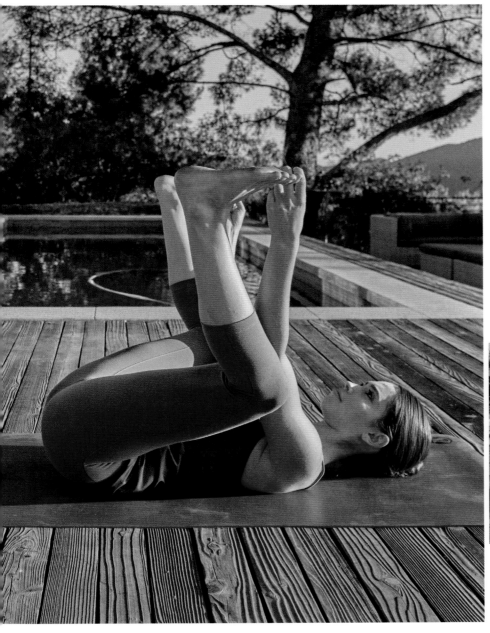

Settle into *stillness*— focusing only on your breath as it *flows* through your nose

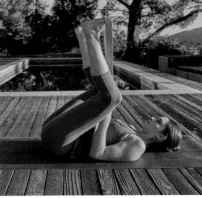

MAKE IT EASIER
In step 3, use a strap around each foot to pull your feet upward.

3 Reach your arms up between your legs and grab your big toes with your fingers. Pull your feet up until the soles of your feet are completely facing upward, keeping your knees bent. Pull your knees toward your chest without lifting your hips or head off the ground. **Hold.** Inhale and exhale slow, steady breaths through your nose. Slowly reverse out of the pose.

Thread the needle

This twisting asana focuses on the thoracic spine, and it's a great preparation for doing backbends. It's also a calming pose that will remove the kinks from your back after a night's sleep or after a long day of standing on your feet.

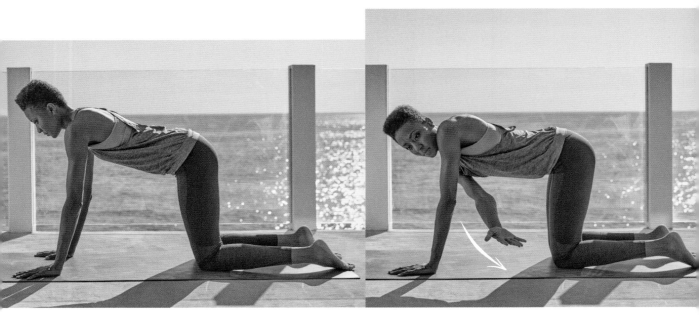

1 Put your hands and knees on the ground, with your hands flat and your fingers pointing forward. Keep your spine and neck parallel to the ground and your eyes looking down.

2 Reach your right arm underneath your body, rotate your upper body at your hips, and turn your head toward your left side.

BE AWARE If you've ever suffered any kind of neck or spine injury, use caution when practicing twists, especially if you feel pain.

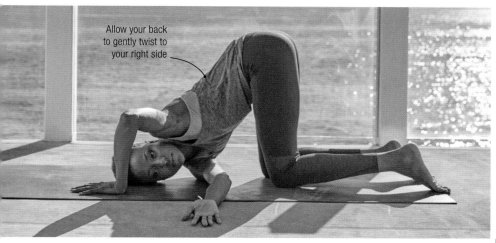

Allow your back
to gently twist to
your right side

Breathe into
your heart—
feel it *expand*
as you inhale
and *soften*
as you exhale

3 Bend your left elbow and lower your right shoulder
and right ear to the ground.

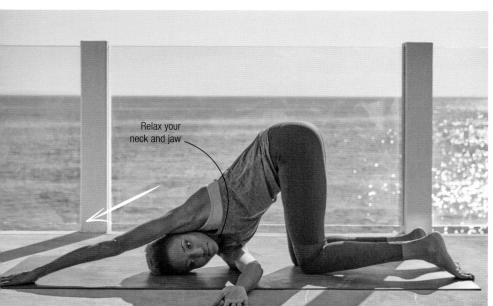

Relax your
neck and jaw

4 Keep your hips aligned with your knees and extend your
left arm forward, keeping your elbow unbent and pressing
your left palm into the ground to open up your upper back.
Hold. Inhale and exhale slow, steady breaths through your
nose. Slowly reverse out of the pose as you return to your
starting position, then repeat with the opposite arm.

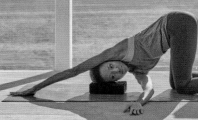

MAKE IT EASIER
In steps 3 and 4, place
your head on a block
to provide support for
your neck.

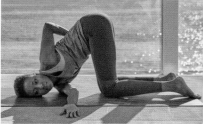

MAKE IT HARDER
In step 3, bend your
left elbow and put
your left hand behind
your lower back.

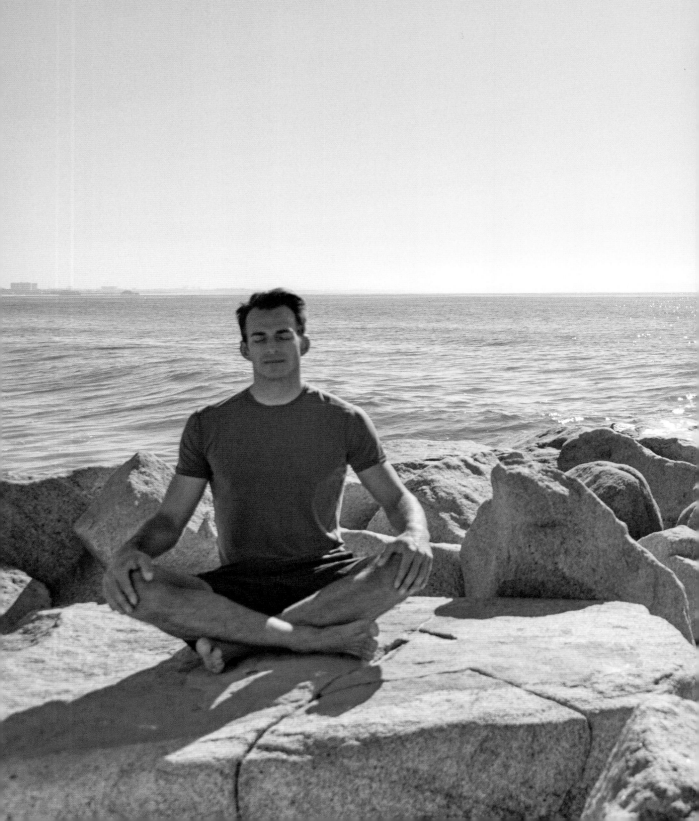

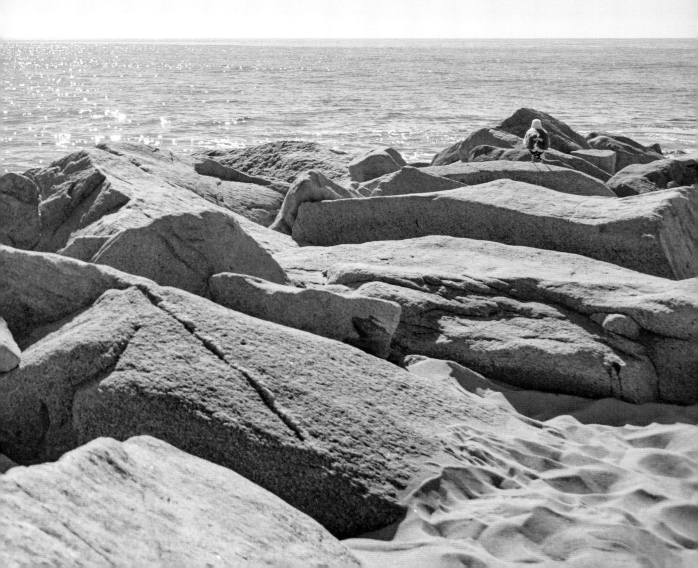

"Remember, it doesn't matter how *deep into a posture* you go— what does matter is *who you are* when you get there"

Max Strom

Bowtie

This asana provides a deep shoulder stretch using your own body weight to get into position. It's a calming pose that will help you open up your upper back, which can improve posture by counteracting the rounding that occurs while sitting at a desk.

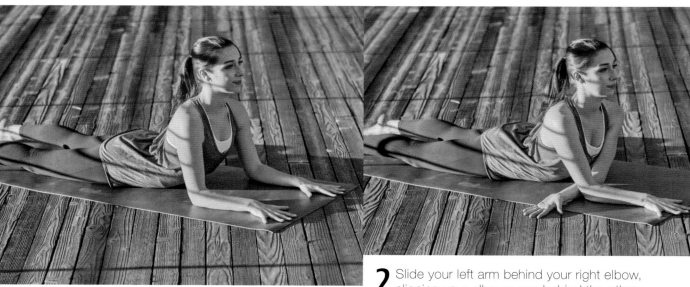

1 Lie on your stomach, with your legs fully extended behind you, bend your elbows at 90-degree angles, and place your hands flat on the ground in front of you. Lift your head and chest off the ground.

2 Slide your left arm behind your right elbow, aligning your elbows one behind the other. Turn your left palm face up and press your forearms into the ground.

BE AWARE If you've ever suffered any kind of rotator cuff injury, you should avoid this pose because it could aggravate that condition.

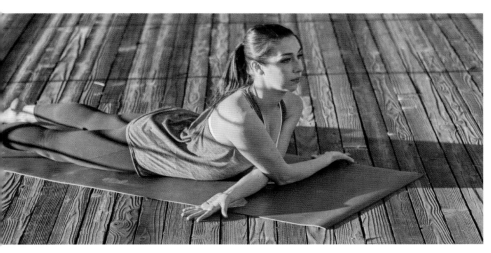

3 Turn your right arm so it slides in the opposite direction from your left arm, continuing to align your elbows. Keep your right hand flat on the ground and continue to press your forearms into the ground.

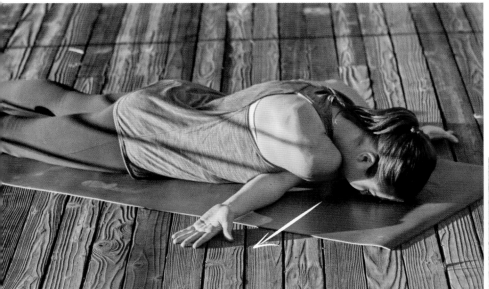

Internally repeat *"I am"* as you inhale and *"at peace"* as you exhale

4 Extend your arms as far away from each other as you can. Lean forward until your forehead touches the ground and your chest rests on top of your folded arms, letting gravity pull you down. **Hold.** Inhale and exhale slow, steady breaths through your nose. Slowly reverse out of the pose /as you return to your starting position, then switch the arm positions and repeat.

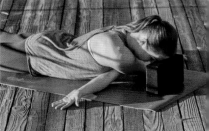

MAKE IT EASIER
In step 4, place a block or a bolster under your head to keep your chest elevated.

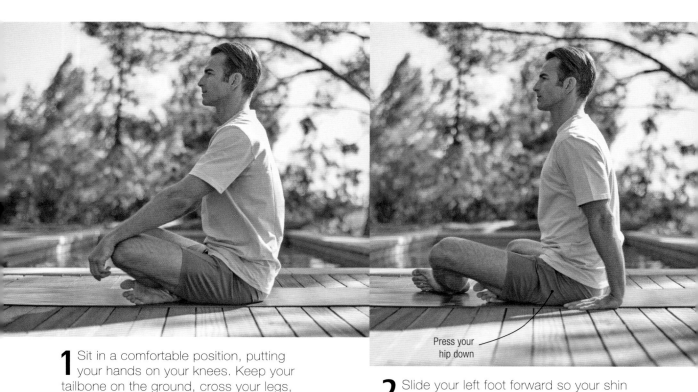

1 Sit in a comfortable position, putting your hands on your knees. Keep your tailbone on the ground, cross your legs, and extend the crown of your head upward.

Press your hip down

2 Slide your left foot forward so your shin is roughly parallel to the top of your mat. (If you feel discomfort in your left knee, keep the heel of your left foot closer to your groin.)

Deer

This unique hip-opening asana combines inner and outer hip rotation to create balance in your hip joints. By adding a twist, this pose might also stimulate digestion, relieve bloating, and soothe lower-back discomfort.

BE AWARE If you have knee pain or have ever suffered any kind of knee injury, place a folded blanket under your front knee.

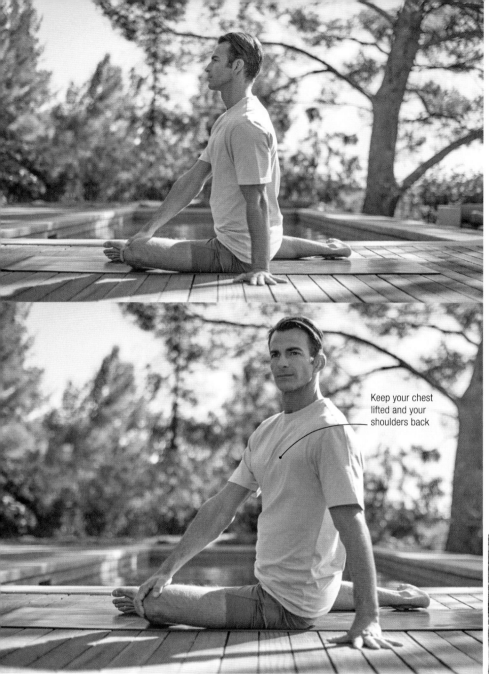

3 Rotate your right foot out and extend your right leg behind you until your right shin is parallel to the side of the mat. Place your right hand on your left knee and your left hand flat on the ground for support.

Internally repeat *"I am enough"* as you hold this pose— let that statement *sink in*

Keep your chest lifted and your shoulders back

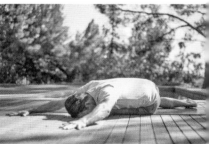

MAKE IT HARDER
In step 4, fold toward the side of your front leg. You can place a bolster under your chest for additional support.

4 Press down into your left hip to keep it close to the ground and lift up through your spine. Move into the twist by gently rotating your chest and shoulders toward your left side. **Hold.** Inhale and exhale slow, steady breaths through your nose. Slowly reverse out of the pose as you return to your starting position, then repeat with the opposite leg.

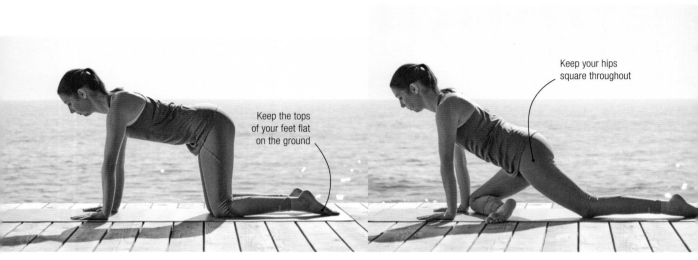

Keep the tops
of your feet flat
on the ground

Keep your hips
square throughout

1 Put your hands and knees on the ground, with your hands flat and your fingers pointing forward. Keep your spine and neck parallel to the ground and your eyes looking down.

2 Slide your right foot forward and underneath your body until your right knee reaches your right wrist, making your leg almost parallel with the top of the mat. Keep the outer side of your right foot flat on the ground.

Swan

This classic asana opens your hips through outer hip rotation— but it requires minimal effort to perform. This pose can also provide relief for lower-body pain. Let gravity do most of the work for you, allowing your body to benefit even more.

BE AWARE If you have knee problems or limited hip mobility, perform the Seated swan (page 114) and Sleeping swan (page 116) instead.

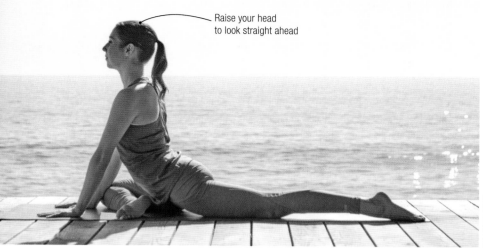

Raise your head
to look straight ahead

3 Fully extend your left leg behind you and lower your hips to the ground, keeping the top of your left foot flat on the ground.

Think about how calm you begin to feel as you breathe deeply

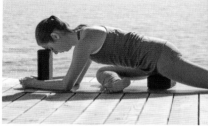

MAKE IT EASIER
In step 3, put a block flat on the ground under your right hip. In step 4, put a block on its short side under your forehead.

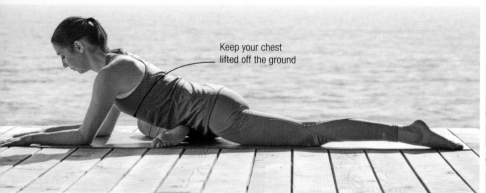

Keep your chest
lifted off the ground

4 Walk your hands forward until your forearms and elbows are flat on the ground. **Hold.** Inhale and exhale slow, steady breaths through your nose. Slowly reverse out of the pose as you return to your starting position, then repeat with the opposite leg.

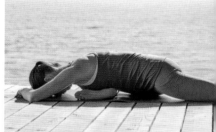

MAKE IT HARDER
In step 3, slide your right leg to an even more perpendicular position to your body. In step 4, lean forward far enough to put your head on the ground.

Seated swan

This asana promotes hip flexibility and takes a more cautious approach with your knees than the classic Swan pose while still engaging your upper body. It can also relieve sciatica pain and can help improve your posture.

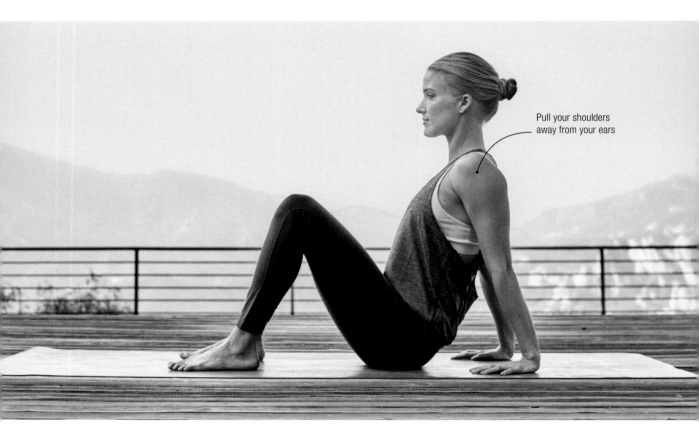

Pull your shoulders away from your ears

1 Sit on the ground, bend your knees, and put your feet flat on the ground. Place your hands behind you for support, with your fingers pointing forward.

BE AWARE If you've ever suffered lower-back problems, use caution while performing this asana.

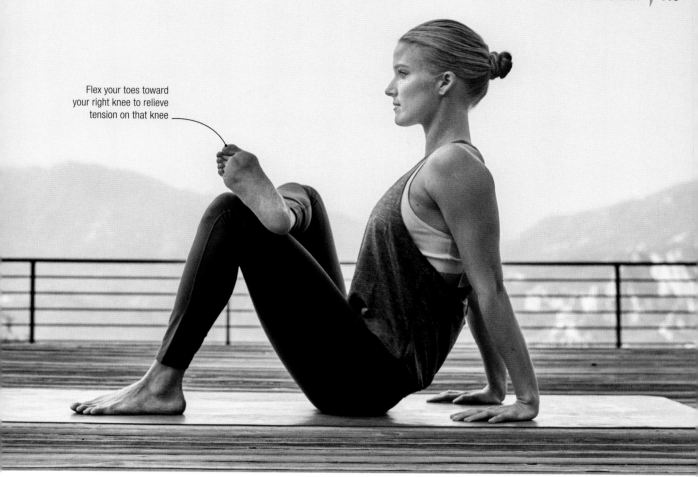

Flex your toes toward your right knee to relieve tension on that knee

2 Slowly bring your right foot over your left knee and rest your right ankle just above your left knee. Gently push your right knee away from your body. **Hold.** Inhale and exhale slow, steady breaths through your nose. Slowly reverse out of the pose as you return to your starting position, then repeat with the opposite leg.

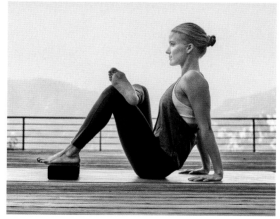

MAKE IT EASIER
In step 2, place a bolster or block under the foot that remains on the ground.

Sleeping swan

This is a more challenging version of the classic Swan asana. It will help you reach and improve the same muscles and tissues as that pose—including your hips, groin, glutes, and lower back—while reducing pressure on your knees.

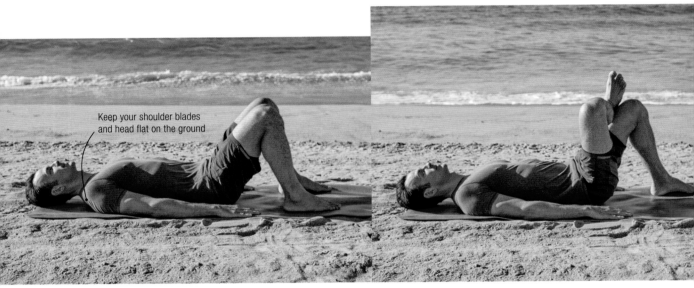

Keep your shoulder blades and head flat on the ground

1 Lie on your back and bend your knees, with your feet flat on the ground. Relax your arms at your sides and keep your hands flat on the ground.

2 Slowly bring your right foot over your left knee and rest your right ankle just above your left knee. Flex your right toes toward your right knee to relieve tension on that knee and gently push your right knee away from your body.

BE AWARE If you've ever suffered any neck or shoulder problems, use caution when performing this asana.

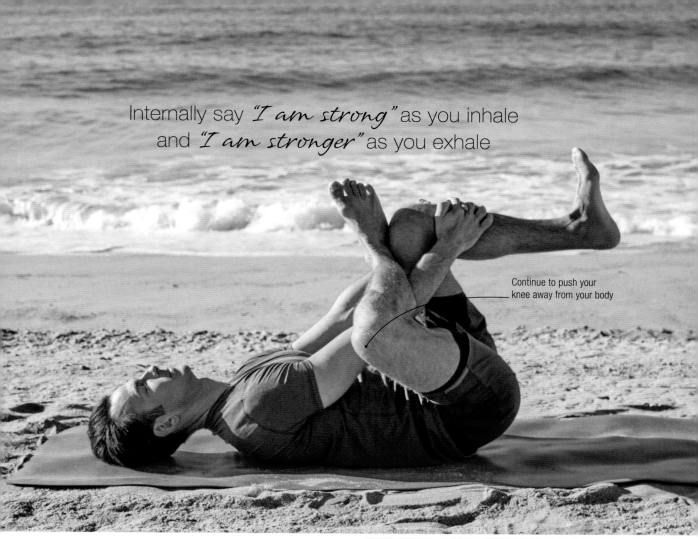

Internally say *"I am strong"* as you inhale
and *"I am stronger"* as you exhale

Continue to push your
knee away from your body

3 Reach your right arm through the opening
between your legs and reach your left arm
around the outside of your left leg. Intertwine your
fingers just below your left knee and pull your left
thigh toward your stomach. **Hold.** Inhale and
exhale slow, steady breaths through your nose.
Slowly reverse out of the pose as you return to
your starting position, then repeat with the
opposite leg.

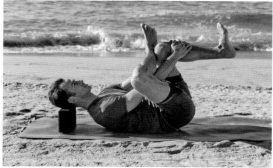

MAKE IT EASIER
In step 1, place a bolster or a block
under your head.

Child's pose

In addition to stretching your back muscles, this classic asana calms your nerves and encourages the relaxation of your body and mind. It's a wonderful pose to do when you need to unwind after a long day.

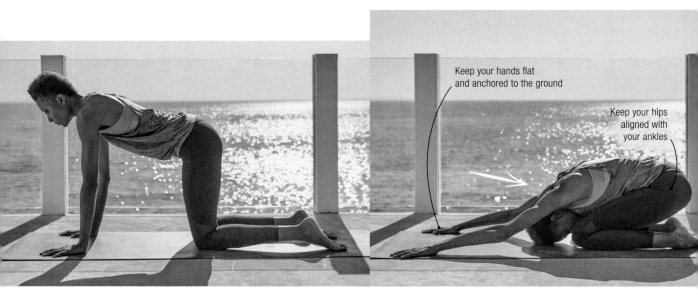

Keep your hands flat and anchored to the ground

Keep your hips aligned with your ankles

1 Place your hands and knees on the ground, with your hands flat and your fingers pointing forward. Keep your spine and neck parallel to the ground and your eyes looking down.

2 Bring your feet together until your big toes touch. Push your hips back and down, bringing them as close to your heels as possible, and rest your head on the ground.

BE AWARE If you have sensitive knees, you might find this pose uncomfortable and should perform the Reclined child's pose (page 120) instead.

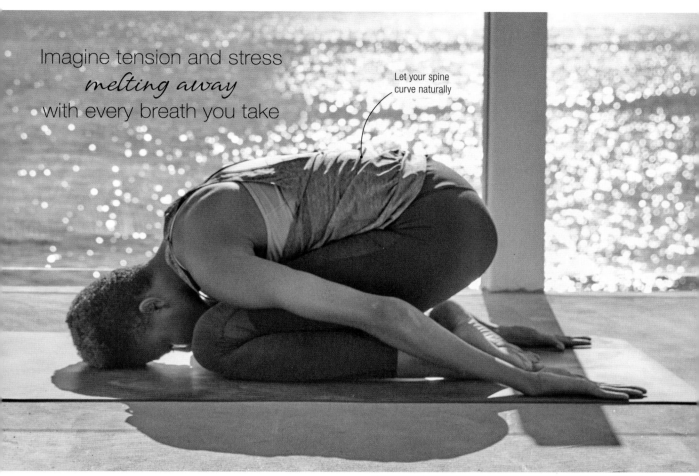

Imagine tension and stress *melting away* with every breath you take

Let your spine curve naturally

3 Extend your arms toward the back of your mat, turning your palms upward and keeping the backs of your hands flat on the ground. Let your shoulders rest on your knees. **Hold.** Inhale and exhale slow, steady breaths through your nose. Slowly reverse out of the pose.

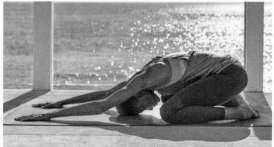

MAKE IT EASIER
In step 2, widen the space between your knees and extend your arms farther forward.

Reclined child's pose

This asana offers the same benefits as the traditional Child's pose, but it's easier on your knees. It's a restorative and meditative pose you can do anytime you feel stressed.

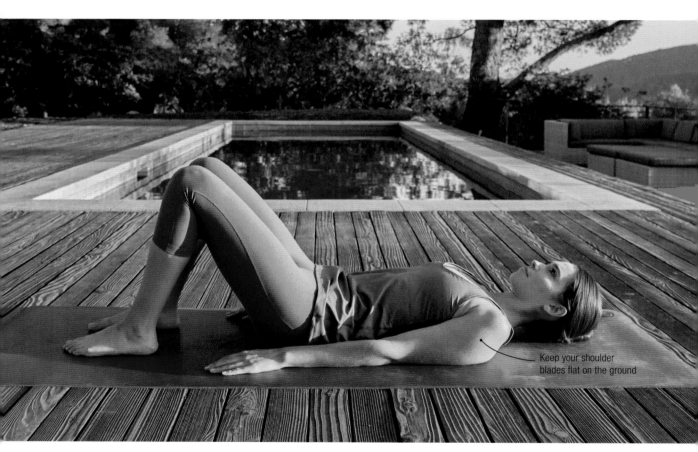

Keep your shoulder
blades flat on the ground

1 Lie on your back and bend your knees, with your feet flat on the ground and your knees together. Relax your arms at your sides and keep your hands flat on the ground.

BE AWARE If lying flat on your back feels or becomes uncomfortable, you can place a pillow under your head to support your neck.

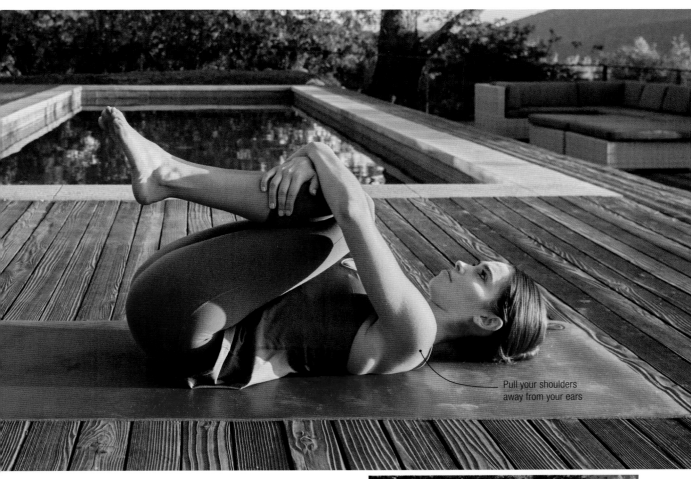

Pull your shoulders
away from your ears

2 Bring your knees toward your chest, wrap your
arms around your knees, and position each
hand just below its opposite knee. Keep your
head and shoulders on the ground, but lift your
tailbone off the ground. **Hold.** Inhale and exhale
slow, steady breaths through your nose. Slowly
reverse out of the pose.

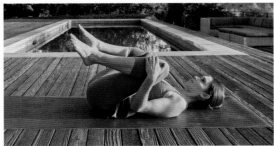

MAKE IT HARDER
In step 2, widen your knees, place your hands
on your knees, and press your tailbone down.

When you *inhale*,
lengthen your spine,
and when you *exhale*,
pull your knees closer

Cat pulling its tail

This advanced asana combines a reclining twist with a slight backbend. It also stretches your iliotibial (IT) band and quadriceps to restore and revitalize your entire body, including relieving stiffness in your lower back.

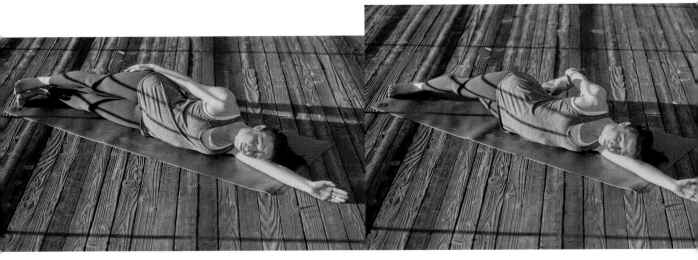

1 Lie on your left side, extending your left arm toward the top of your mat and placing your head on your arm. Place your right hand flat on the side of your right thigh and stack your right leg on top of your left leg.

2 Bend your left knee and reach your right arm behind you to grab the inside of your left foot with your right hand. Press your left heel out and away from your glutes, but keep your hips aligned.

BE AWARE If you have a sensitive lower back or have ever suffered any kind of lower-back injury, you might want to avoid this pose.

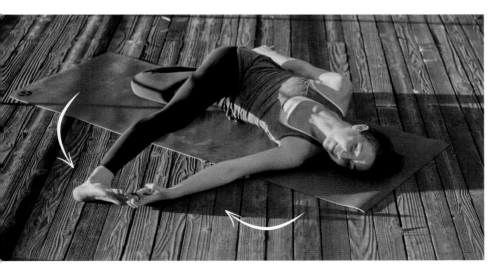

3 Slide your right leg out toward the left side of your mat until it's parallel with the bottom of your mat. Reach your left hand out to grab your right big toe. Keep your head flat on the ground.

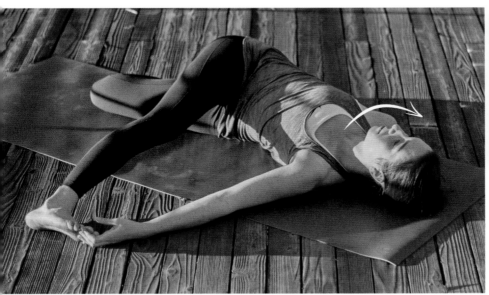

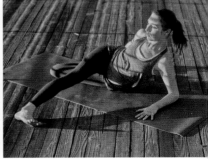

MAKE IT EASIER
In step 3, prop yourself on your left forearm and let your right leg go out to the side on its own. Keep holding your left foot with your right hand. In step 4, hold this position.

4 Move into a spinal twist by dropping your right shoulder toward the ground and keeping your right hip stacked over your left hip as much as possible. **Hold.** Inhale and exhale slow, steady breaths through your nose. Slowly reverse out of the pose as you return to your starting position, then repeat with the opposite leg.

Supported fish

This restorative asana connects with your heart chakra and helps balance your energy levels. It also invites you to breathe deeply into your chest and stretches the muscles around your rib cage. You'll need two blocks for this pose.

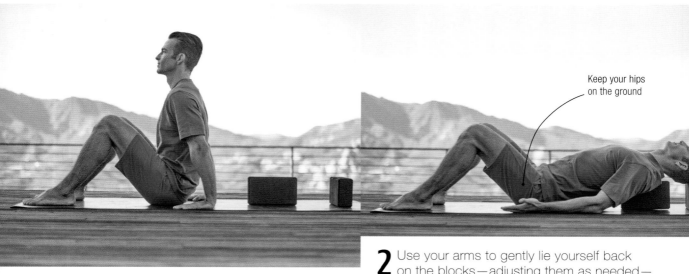

Keep your hips on the ground

1 Place two blocks on their long sides behind you—one placed lengthwise for your upper back and one placed perpendicular for your head. Sit on the ground, bending your knees and keeping your feet flat on the ground, with your hands behind you and your fingers pointing forward.

2 Use your arms to gently lie yourself back on the blocks—adjusting them as needed—so your upper back, neck, and head are supported. Position your arms at your sides, with your hands flat on the ground and your palms facing up.

BE AWARE If you've ever suffered any kind of back injury, use caution when doing backbends. Go slowly—and stop if you experience any pain.

Internally repeat the affirmation
"I am open and receptive to love"

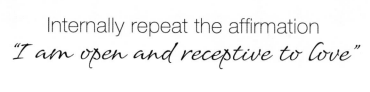

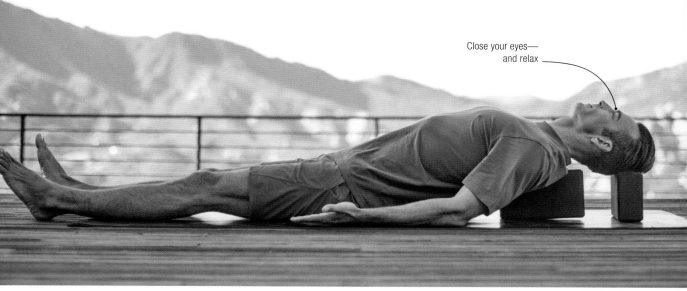

Close your eyes—
and relax

3 Extend your legs out in front of you to allow your hips and lower back to settle into the ground. **Hold.** Inhale and exhale slow, steady breaths through your nose. Slowly reverse out of the pose.

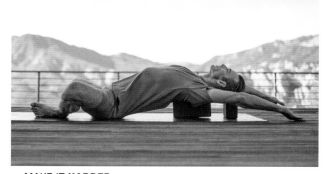

MAKE IT HARDER
In step 3, reach your arms over your head, touching the ground with the backs of your fingers. Push your bent knees outward to bring the soles of your feet together.

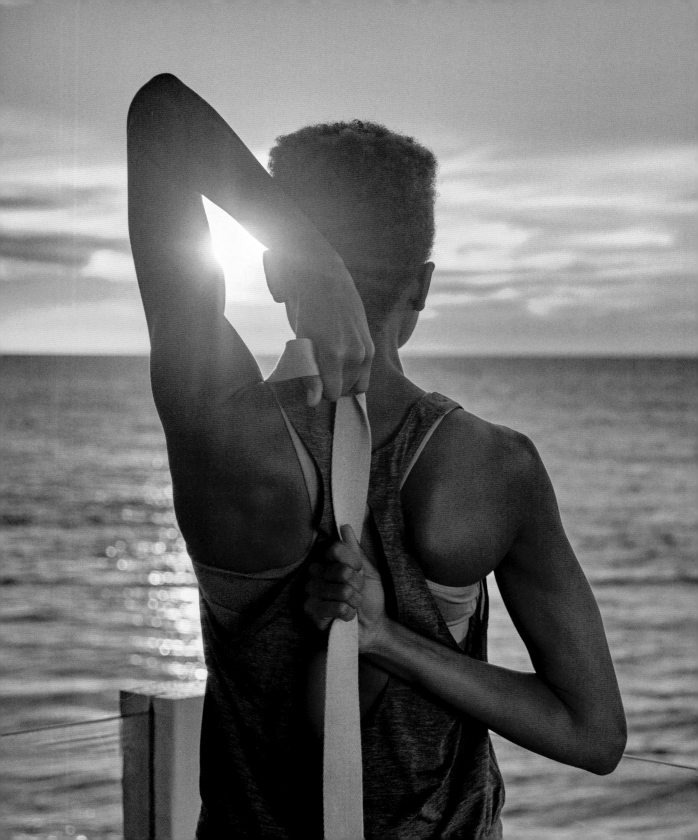

"Change yourself—*you are in control*"

Mahatma Gandhi

Melting heart

As its name suggests, this asana opens up the area near your heart by stretching deeply into your shoulders and the muscles around your rib cage. It might also help soothe and relax your nerves.

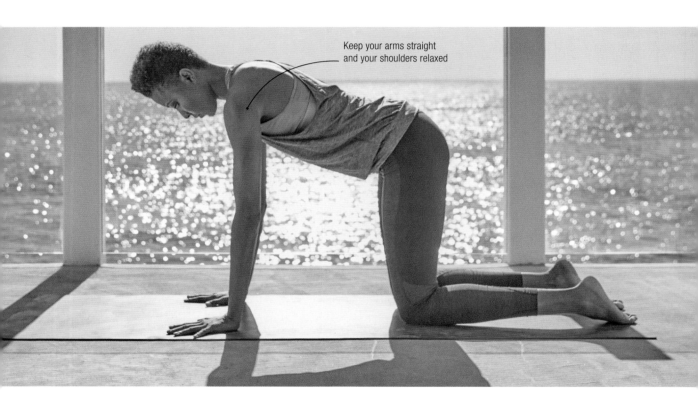

Keep your arms straight and your shoulders relaxed

1 Put your hands and knees on the ground, with your hands flat and your fingers pointing forward. Keep your spine and neck parallel to the ground and your eyes looking down.

BE AWARE If you have sensitive knees, place a folded blanket underneath them. If you've suffered any kind of neck injury, you might find this pose uncomfortable.

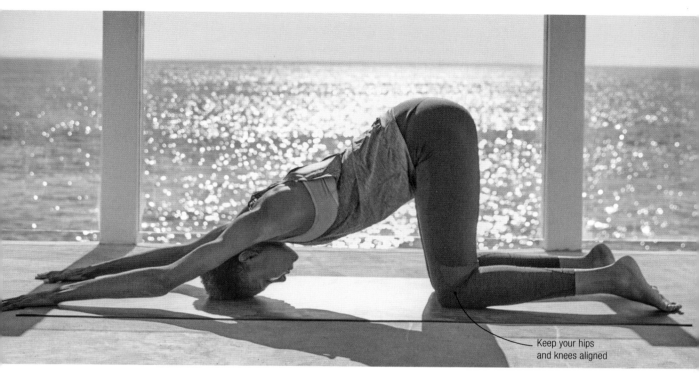

Keep your hips
and knees aligned

2 Walk your hands out in front of you until you can lower
your forehead to the ground. Reach through your arms,
soften your neck and upper back, and feel your rib cage
expand. **Hold.** Inhale and exhale slow, steady breaths
through your nose. Slowly reverse out of the pose.

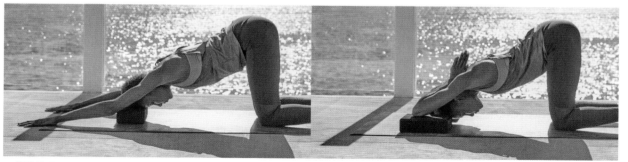

MAKE IT EASIER
In step 2, if your forehead can't touch the ground,
place a block underneath it for support.

MAKE IT HARDER
In step 2, place one block under each elbow
to elevate your arms. Press your hands together
and bend your elbows so your hands rest on the
back of your head. This allows you to go deeper
into the pose to stretch your triceps.

Legs up the wall

This beginner-friendly asana is the perfect pose to do after a long day of standing on your feet or following a vigorous workout. This mild inversion will help soothe and restore aching legs and prepare you for deep sleep.

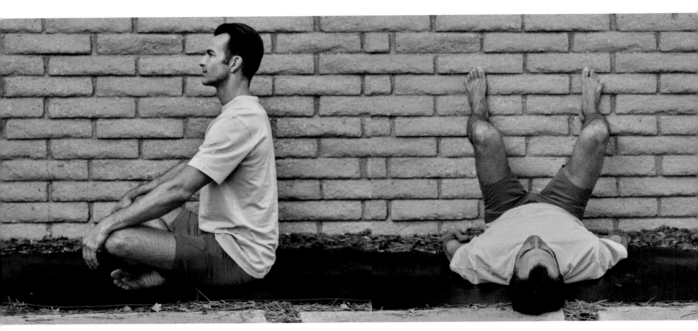

1 Sit in a comfortable position 6 inches (15cm) away from a wall, facing your right side toward the wall and putting your hands on your knees. Keep your tailbone on the ground, cross your legs, and extend the crown of your head upward.

2 Gently lie on your back, rotating your body until your tailbone faces the wall. Rest the bottom of your feet flat on the wall and bend your knees toward your stomach. Relax your head and neck.

BE AWARE Because inversions can increase the pressure around your eyes, this isn't a good pose for anyone suffering from glaucoma.

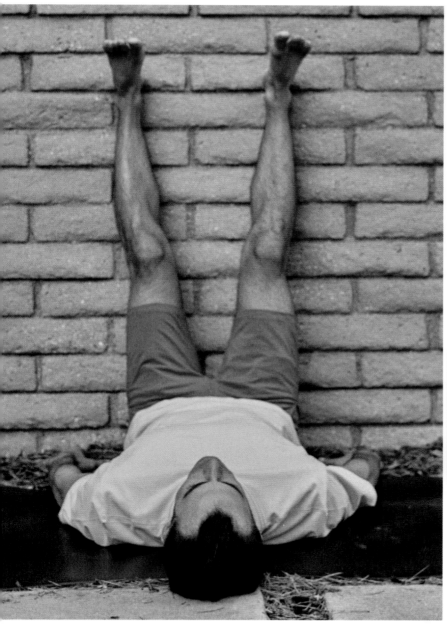

Think *"I am"*
as you inhale
and *"at ease"*
as you exhale

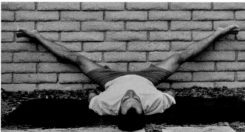

MAKE IT HARDER
In step 3, bring your hips
closer to the wall and widen
your legs as far as possible.

3 Fully extend your legs upward to rest your heels against the wall, keeping a slight bend in your knees to prevent hyperextending them. **Hold.** Inhale and exhale slow, steady breaths through your nose. Slowly reverse out of the pose.

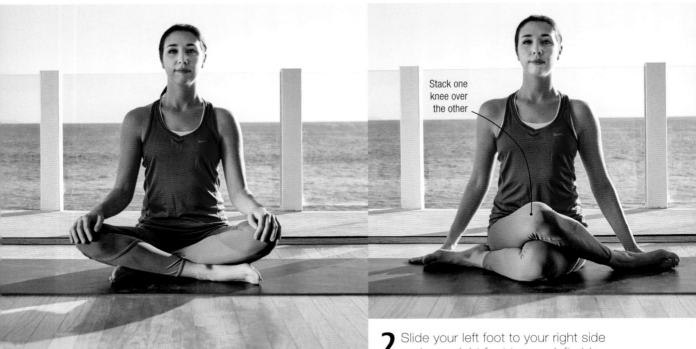

Stack one
knee over
the other

1 Sit in a comfortable position, with your hands on your knees. Keep your tailbone on the ground, cross your legs, and extend the crown of your head upward.

2 Slide your left foot to your right side and your right foot to your left side until your knees are aligned. Pull your feet toward your hips and place your hands flat on the ground behind you for support.

Shoelace

This seated asana combines the benefits of hip openers and forward folds to help you decompress and unwind when you're feeling stressed or distraught. This might help relieve lower-back pain and soothe your nervous system.

BE AWARE If you have limited hip flexibility, perform the Reclined shoelace (page 134) instead.

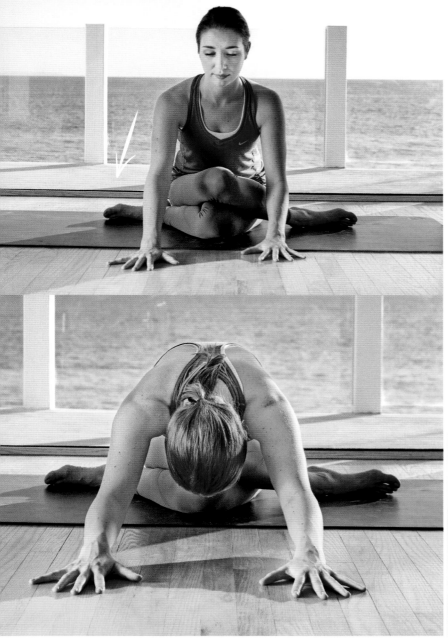

3 Walk your hands out in front of you, slightly bending your elbows, to initiate the forward fold.

If your mind wanders, bring your awareness back to your breath

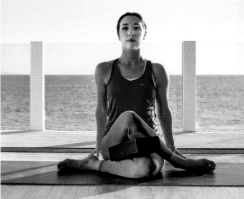

4 Straighten your arms, spread your fingers wide, and fold forward until you find your edge, keeping your tailbone anchored to the ground. **Hold.** Inhale and exhale slow, steady breaths through your nose. Slowly reverse out of the pose as you return to your starting position, then repeat with the opposite leg.

MAKE IT EASIER
In step 2, place a folded blanket or a block between your knees for extra support. In step 4, you can also place a bolster under your chest.

Reclined shoelace

This milder version of the Shoelace asana targets your outer hip without placing too much pressure on your joints. It might also offer relief if you suffer from sciatica.

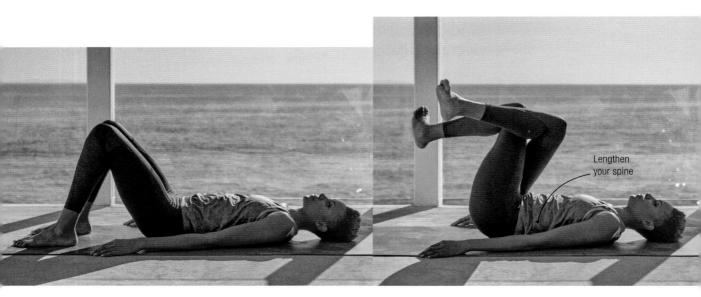

Lengthen your spine

1 Lie on your back and bend your knees, with your feet flat on the ground. Relax your arms at your sides and keep your hands flat on the ground.

2 Lift your legs off the ground and cross your right calf over your left knee, aligning your knees as much as possible. Lightly flex your feet toward your knees.

BE AWARE If you've ever suffered any kind of knee injury, you might find this uncomfortable. When practicing this asana, keep your feet flexed to maintain integrity in your knee joints.

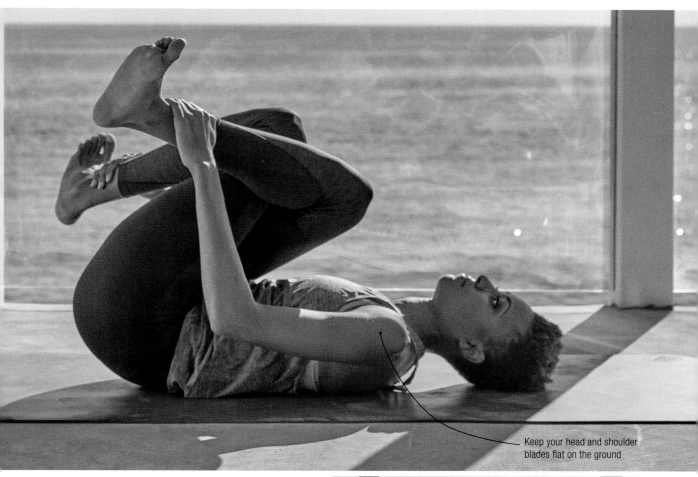

Keep your head and shoulder
blades flat on the ground

3 Grasp your ankles with your hands
and bend your elbows to pull your
legs closer to your stomach. **Hold.** Inhale
and exhale slow, steady breaths through
your nose. Slowly reverse out of the pose
as you return to your starting position,
then repeat with the opposite leg.

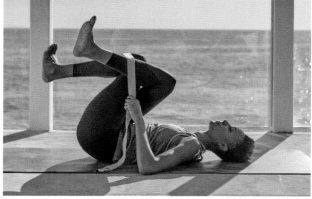

MAKE IT EASIER
In step 3, wrap a strap around your shins.

Reverse prayer arms

This upper-body asana is a great way to stretch your wrists and relieve aches and pains after working at a computer. This pose also opens up your chest and shoulders to promote good posture.

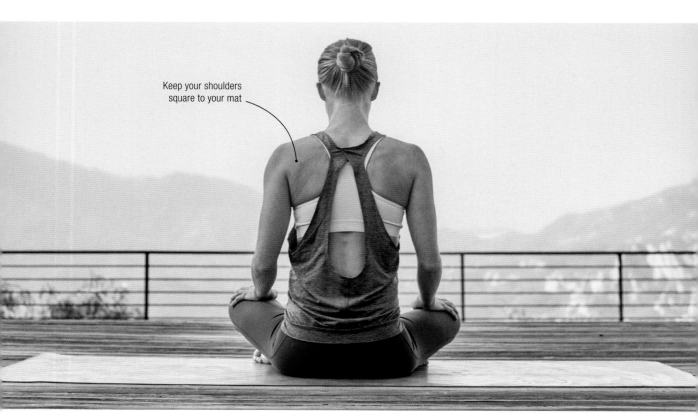

Keep your shoulders square to your mat

1 Sit in a comfortable position, with your hands on your knees. Keep your tailbone on the ground, cross your legs, and extend the crown of your head upward.

BE AWARE If you've ever suffered any kind of rotator cuff or wrist injury, you might want to avoid this pose, especially if it causes pain.

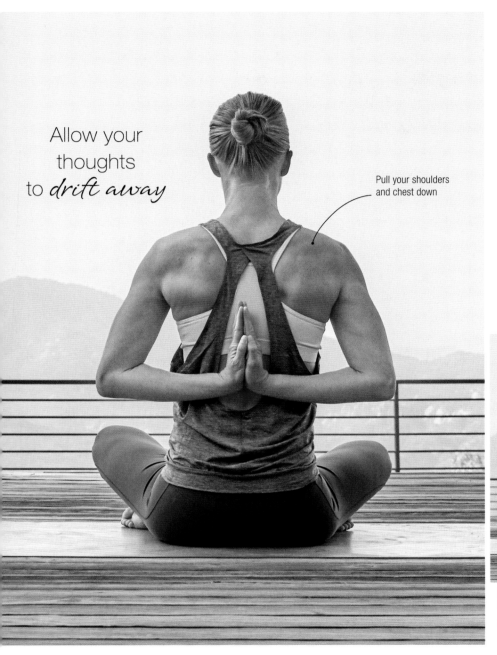

Allow your
thoughts
to *drift away*

Pull your shoulders
and chest down

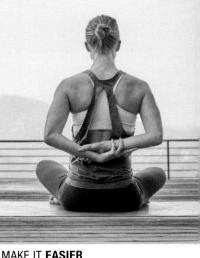

MAKE IT EASIER
In step 2, wrap your hands
around your wrists.

2 Reach your arms behind your back, bending your elbows,
and press your palms and fingers together, with your
fingertips pointing up. **Hold.** Inhale and exhale slow, steady
breaths through your nose. Slowly reverse out of the pose.

Frog

This simple yet intense asana will help you open up your inner thighs and groin to improve hip flexibility. You'll need two blankets for this pose.

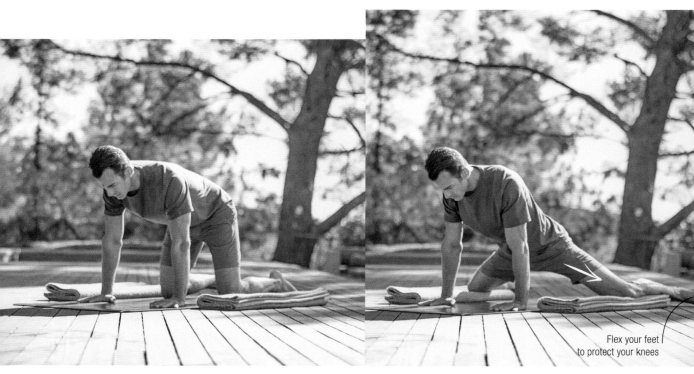

Flex your feet
to protect your knees

1 Place a folded blanket on each side of your mat. Place your hands and knees on the ground, with your hands flat and your fingers pointing forward. Keep your spine and neck parallel to the ground and your eyes looking down.

2 Widen your knees as far as comfortable, making sure they stay aligned with your hips, and place them on the blankets. Align your ankles with your knees and flex your feet so your toes point out to your sides.

BE AWARE If you have tight hips or sensitive knees and ankles, you might find this pose uncomfortable, so use a bolster for added support or perform the Child's pose (page 118) instead.

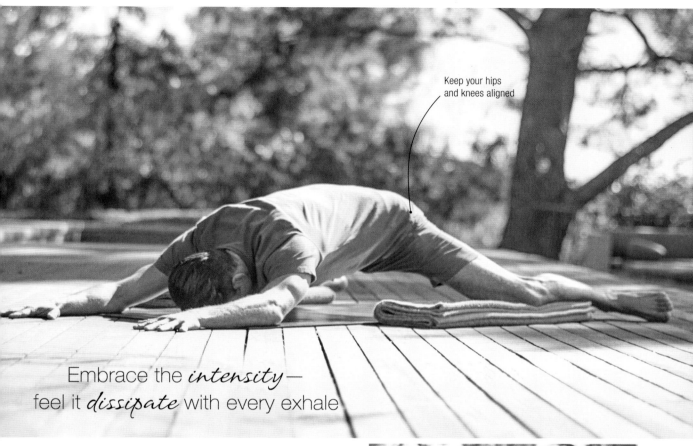

Keep your hips
and knees aligned

Embrace the *intensity*—
feel it *dissipate* with every exhale

3 Without changing the alignment in your lower
body, keep your chest lifted as you bend your
elbows and walk your hands forward until your
forearms, elbows, and forehead touch the ground.
Allow gravity to pull your hips down. **Hold.** Inhale
and exhale slow, steady breaths through your
nose. Slowly reverse out of the pose.

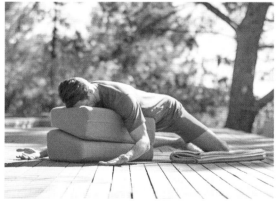

MAKE IT EASIER
In step 3, place a bolster or two under your
upper body and head and angle your legs
to allow you to touch your big toes together.

Half monkey

This asana opens up your hamstrings and prepares you for the full Monkey pose. Runners will especially benefit from this asana because it stretches the hamstrings, groin, and calves.

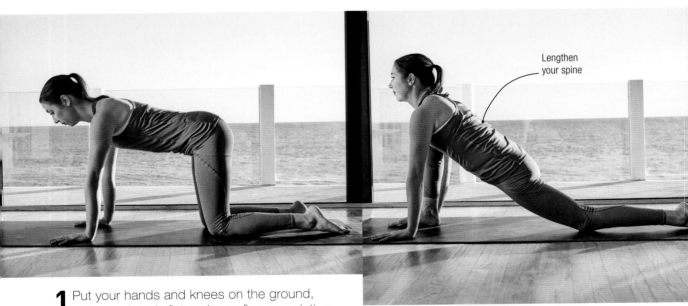

Lengthen your spine

1 Put your hands and knees on the ground, with your hands flat and your fingers pointing forward. Keep your spine and neck parallel to the ground and your eyes looking down.

2 Step your right foot forward toward the top corner of your mat and positioned to the inside of your right hand, aligning your right knee directly over your right ankle.

BE AWARE If you've ever suffered any kind of groin or hamstring tear, use caution during this pose because it could aggravate either condition.

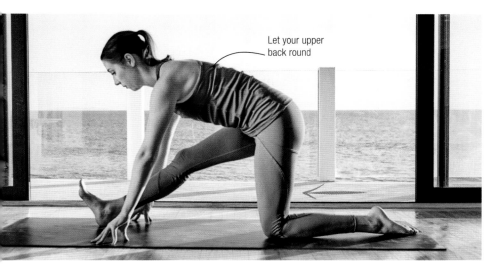

Let your upper
back round

3 Straighten your right leg and shift your hips back until
they align over your left knee. Walk your hands forward
on your fingertips until your fingers align with your right
ankle. Keep the top of your left foot flat on the ground
and your right leg supported on the heel of your right foot.

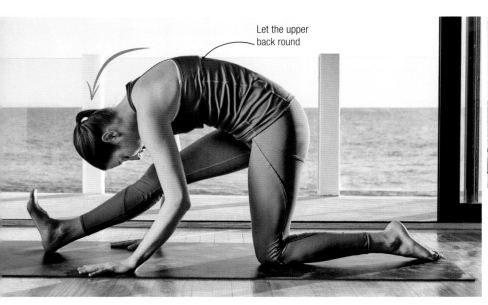

Let the upper
back round

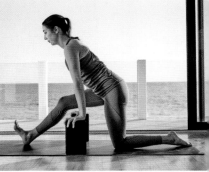

MAKE IT EASIER
In step 3, place a block
under each palm and
keep your chest elevated.
You can also slightly
bend your front knee.

4 Place your hands flat on the ground and fold forward toward
your right knee. **Hold.** Inhale and exhale slow, steady breaths
through your nose. Slowly reverse out of the pose as you return
to your starting position, then repeat with the opposite leg.

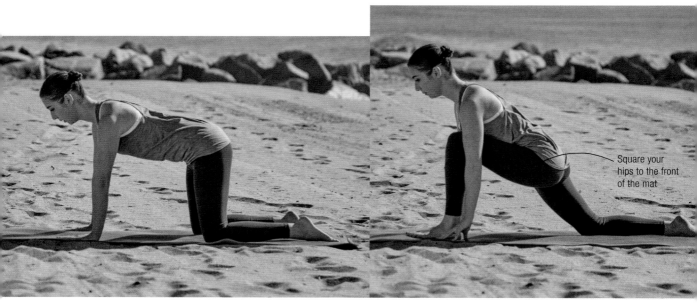

Square your hips to the front of the mat

1 Put your hands and knees on the ground, with your hands flat and your fingers pointing forward. Keep your spine and neck parallel to the ground and your eyes looking down.

2 Step your left foot forward toward the top corner of your mat and positioned to the inside of your left hand, aligning your left knee directly over your left ankle. Align your hands with your left ankle and use your fingertips for balance.

Monkey

This advanced asana is a deep hip opener as well as an intense hamstring stretch. The key is to go into this pose slowly and mindfully but never rushing the process.

BE AWARE If you've ever suffered any kind of groin injury or hamstring tear, use caution because this pose could aggravate either condition.

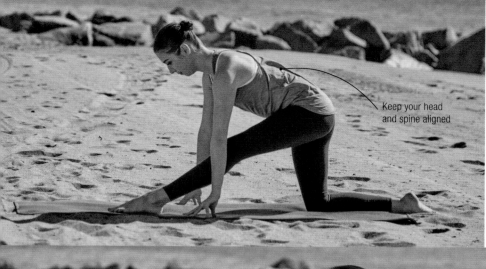

Keep your head
and spine aligned

3 Extend your left foot
forward as far as you
can and shift your hips
back until they align over
your right knee.

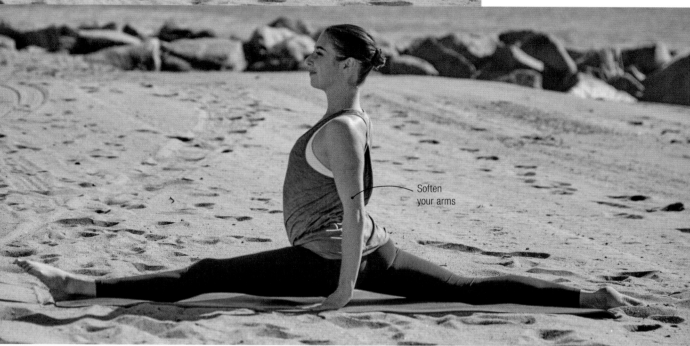

Soften
your arms

4 Extend your right leg behind you, letting
gravity pull your hips down as you put your
hands flat on the ground for support. **Hold.**
Inhale and exhale slow, steady breaths through
your nose. Slowly reverse out of the pose as
you return to your starting position, then switch
the leg positions and repeat.

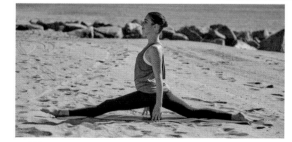

MAKE IT EASIER
In step 4, place a block or a bolster
under your hips.

Corpse

This classic asana is the last pose performed during any yin yoga practice. It's a vital component to any yin yoga sequence because it can rejuvenate your mind and body.

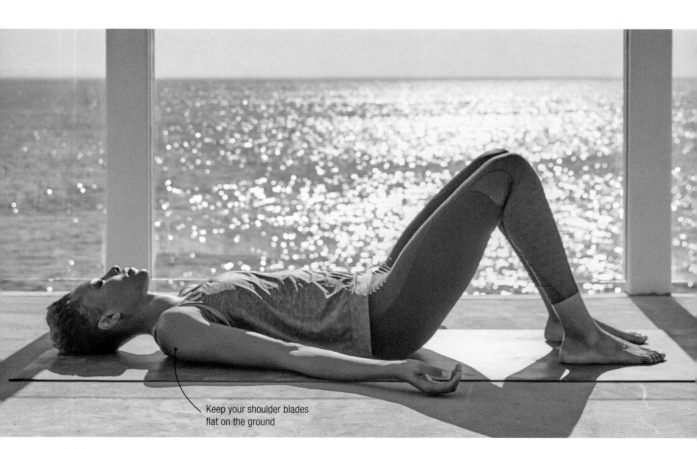

Keep your shoulder blades
flat on the ground

1 Lie on your back and bend your knees, keeping your feet flat on the ground. Relax your arms at your sides, with your fingers curled slightly upward.

As you inhale, picture a *wave of peace* washing over you, and as you exhale, picture the *wave taking away* stress

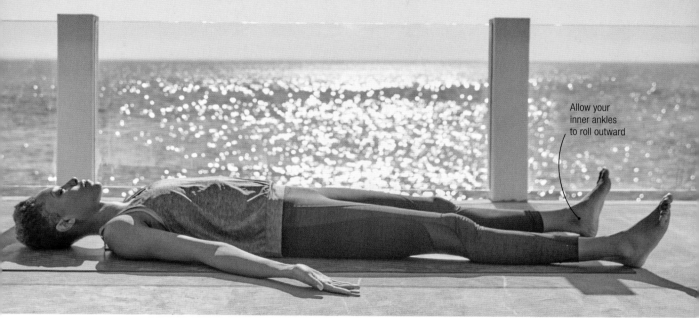

Allow your inner ankles to roll outward

2 Extend your legs out one at a time, placing your heels toward the sides of the mat and letting gravity pull your feet down. Pull your shoulders down from your ears and extend your hands. **Hold.** Inhale and exhale slow, steady breaths through your nose. Slowly reverse out of the pose.

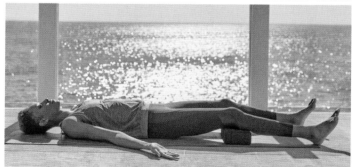

MAKE IT EASIER
In step 2, place a block under each knee.

Yin sequences

Within this chapter you'll practice sequences that combine asanas into unique flows, helping you reach a variety of goals. Ranging from 30 minutes to 90 minutes, these sequences are perfect for yoga beginners and veterans.

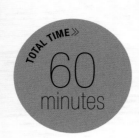

TOTAL TIME »

60
minutes

Pre-workout stretch

This is excellent to do before exercises that actively engage your muscles and elevate your heart rate. This sequence is also good on days between workouts to help your joints heal and recover.

REQUIRED PROP
• 1 blanket

OPTIONAL PROPS
• 2 blocks
• 1 bolster
• 1 strap

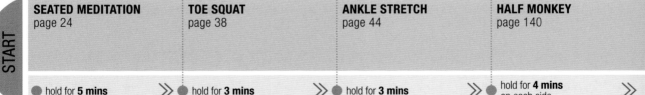

START

SEATED MEDITATION page 24	**TOE SQUAT** page 38	**ANKLE STRETCH** page 44	**HALF MONKEY** page 140
hold for **5 mins**	hold for **3 mins**	hold for **3 mins**	hold for **4 mins** on each side

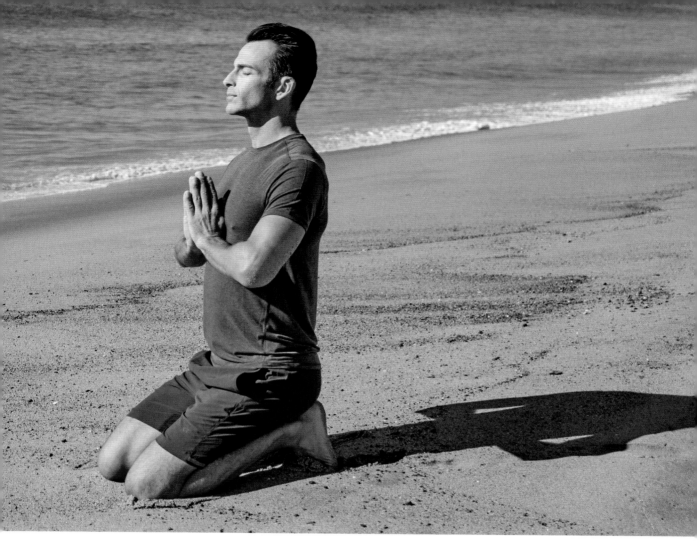

SHOELACE with EAGLE ARMS pages 132 and 100	FROG page 138	SLEEPING SWAN (right side) page 116	IT BAND STRETCH (right side) page 40
hold for **5 mins** on each side	hold for **5 mins**	hold for **5 mins**	hold for **5 mins**

SLEEPING SWAN (left side) page 116	IT BAND STRETCH (left side) page 40	CORPSE page 144	FINISH
hold for **5 mins**	hold for **5 mins**	hold for **6 mins**	

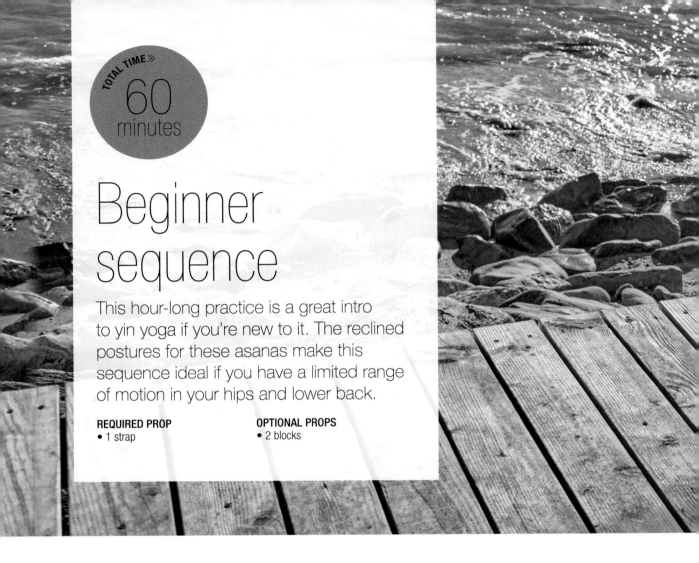

TOTAL TIME »

60
minutes

Beginner sequence

This hour-long practice is a great intro to yin yoga if you're new to it. The reclined postures for these asanas make this sequence ideal if you have a limited range of motion in your hips and lower back.

REQUIRED PROP
• 1 strap

OPTIONAL PROPS
• 2 blocks

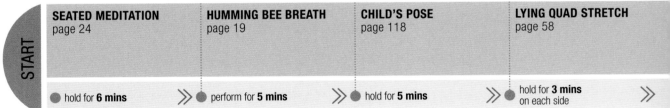

START

SEATED MEDITATION	HUMMING BEE BREATH	CHILD'S POSE	LYING QUAD STRETCH
page 24	page 19	page 118	page 58
● hold for **6 mins**	● perform for **5 mins**	● hold for **5 mins**	● hold for **3 mins** on each side

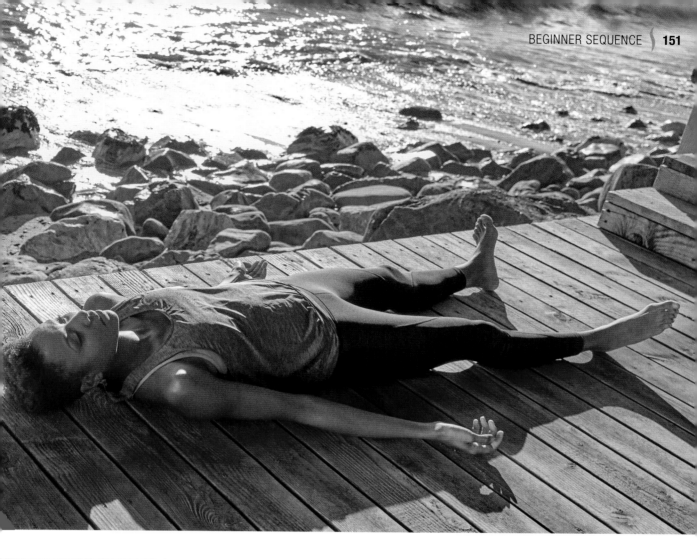

RECLINING LEG STRETCH 1 (right side) page 30	**RECLINING LEG STRETCH 2** (right side) page 32	**RECLINING LEG STRETCH 1** (left side) page 30	**RECLINING LEG STRETCH 2** (left side) page 32
hold for **3 mins**	hold for **3 mins**	hold for **3 mins**	hold for **3 mins**

HALF BUTTERFLY page 52	**RECLINED BUTTERFLY** page 54	**RECLINED CHILD'S POSE** page 120	**CORPSE** page 144	**FINISH**
hold for **5 mins** on each side	hold for **5 mins**	hold for **5 mins**	hold for **6 mins**	

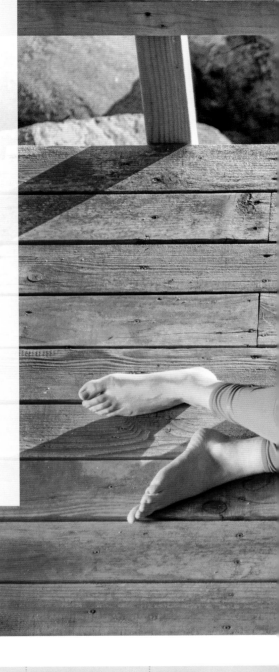

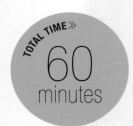

TOTAL TIME »
60
minutes

Improving your digestion

This sequence might provide relief if you're suffering from digestive issues. As you twist and fold forward while performing these asanas, you compress and decompress your stomach, helping stimulate healthy digestion.

REQUIRED PROPS
- none

OPTIONAL PROPS
- block
- bolster
- strap

SEATED MEDITATION
page 24

ALTERNATE NOSTRIL BREATH
page 18

SQUAT
page 36

CATERPILLAR
page 48

SQUARE
page 28

 hold for **6 mins** » hold for **5 mins** » hold for **3 mins** » hold for **5 mins** » hold for **5 mins** on each side »

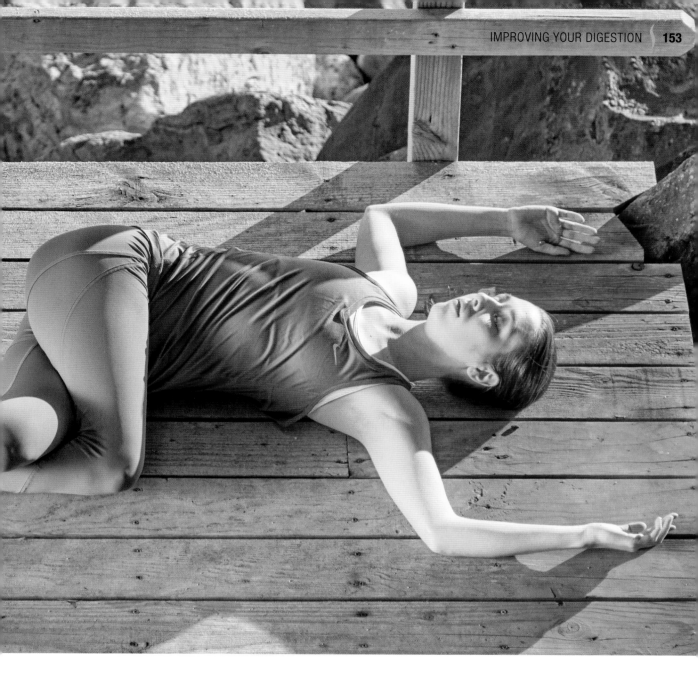

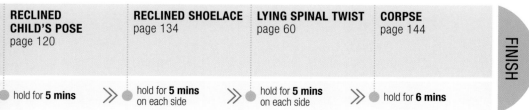

RECLINED CHILD'S POSE
page 120

RECLINED SHOELACE
page 134

LYING SPINAL TWIST
page 60

CORPSE
page 144

FINISH

hold for **5 mins**

hold for **5 mins** on each side

hold for **5 mins** on each side

hold for **6 mins**

Improving your sleep

Indulge in this hour-long practice to prepare for a good night's rest. This sequence uses forward folds and simple reclined poses to help calm your nerves and unwind after a long day. Enjoy a longer rest in the Corpse pose to truly relax and settle down before going to sleep.

REQUIRED PROPS
• none

OPTIONAL PROPS
• 2 blocks

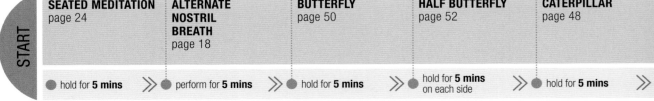

START

SEATED MEDITATION page 24	ALTERNATE NOSTRIL BREATH page 18	BUTTERFLY page 50	HALF BUTTERFLY page 52	CATERPILLAR page 48
hold for **5 mins**	perform for **5 mins**	hold for **5 mins**	hold for **5 mins** on each side	hold for **5 mins**

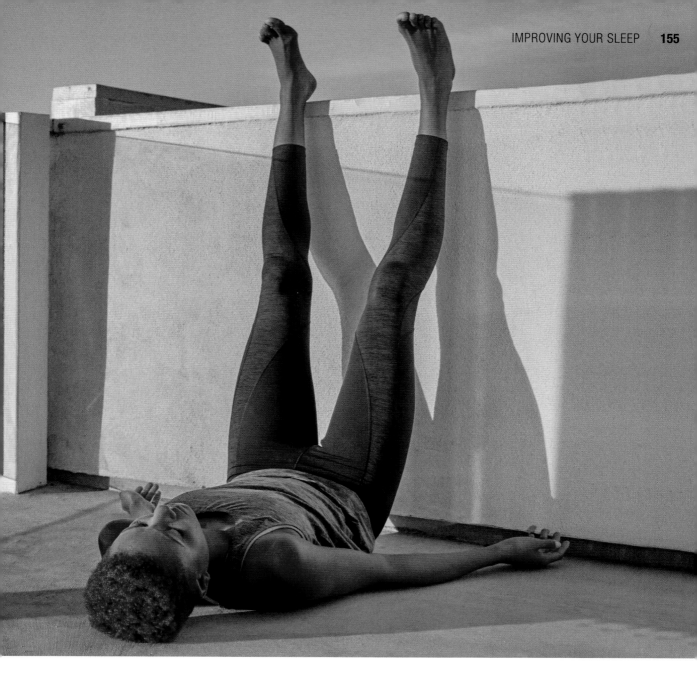

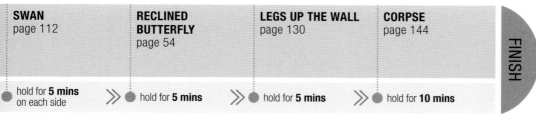

SWAN page 112	RECLINED BUTTERFLY page 54	LEGS UP THE WALL page 130	CORPSE page 144	FINISH
hold for **5 mins** on each side	hold for **5 mins**	hold for **5 mins**	hold for **10 mins**	

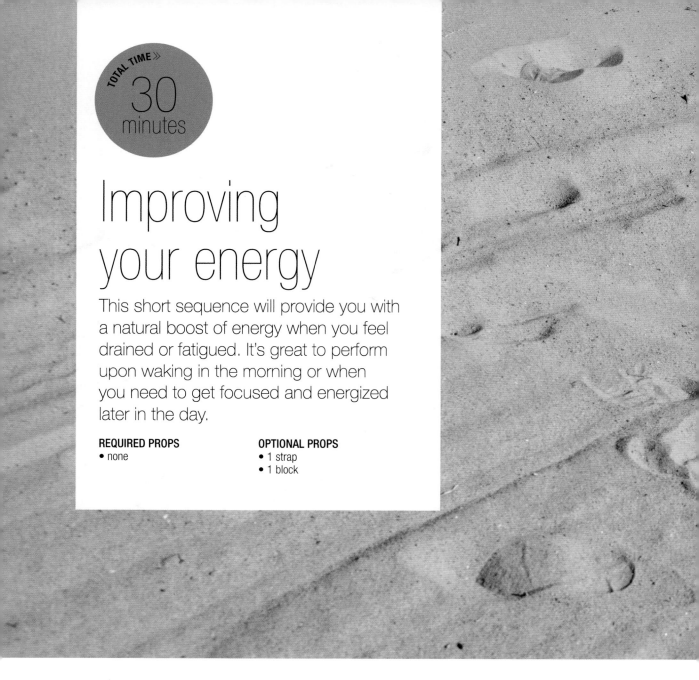

30 minutes

Improving your energy

This short sequence will provide you with a natural boost of energy when you feel drained or fatigued. It's great to perform upon waking in the morning or when you need to get focused and energized later in the day.

REQUIRED PROPS
• none

OPTIONAL PROPS
• 1 strap
• 1 block

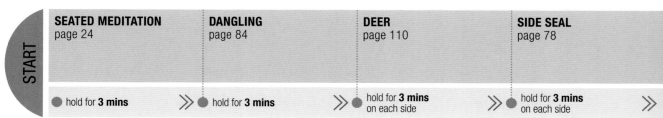

START

SEATED MEDITATION page 24	DANGLING page 84	DEER page 110	SIDE SEAL page 78
● hold for **3 mins**	● hold for **3 mins**	● hold for **3 mins** on each side	● hold for **3 mins** on each side

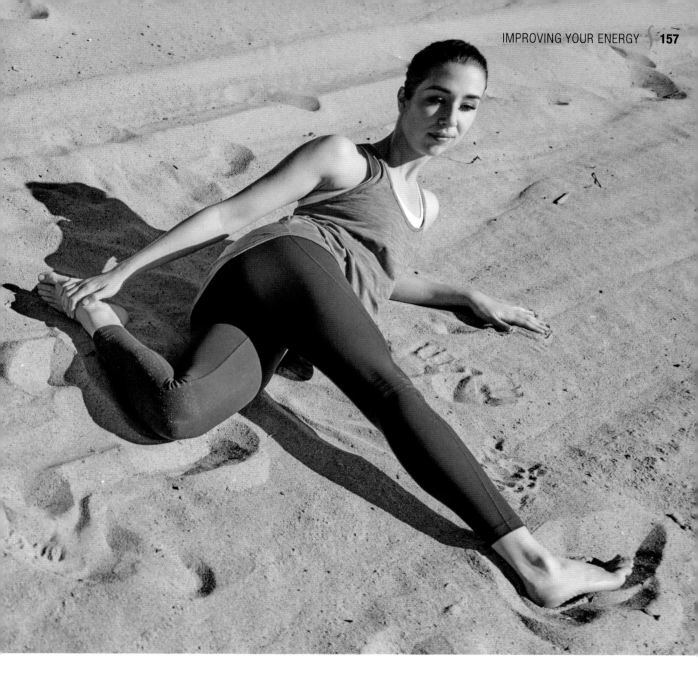

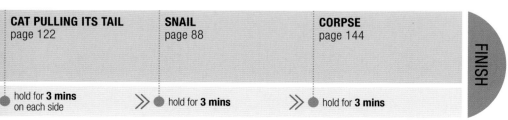

CAT PULLING ITS TAIL page 122	**SNAIL** page 88	**CORPSE** page 144	FINISH
hold for **3 mins** on each side	hold for **3 mins**	hold for **3 mins**	

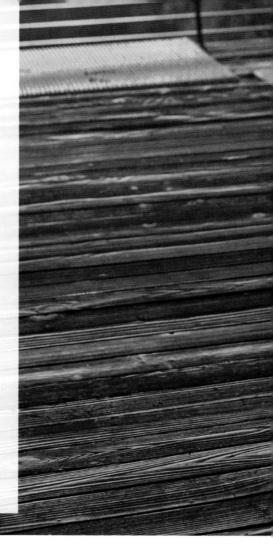

TOTAL TIME »

60
minutes

Intermediate sequence

This hour-long sequence is perfect if you want an overall stretch and already have some flexibility in your hips, hamstrings, and lower back. Focus on the flow of your breath and the tension releasing from your joints as you hold the poses.

REQUIRED PROP
• 1 strap

OPTIONAL PROPS
• 1 additional strap
• 2 blocks

START

SEATED MEDITATION	ALTERNATE NOSTRIL BREATH	REVERSE PRAYER ARMS with TOE SQUAT	WINGED DRAGON
page 24	page 18	pages 136 and 38	page 96
hold for **5 mins**	perform for **5 mins**	hold for **5 mins**	hold for **5 mins** on each side

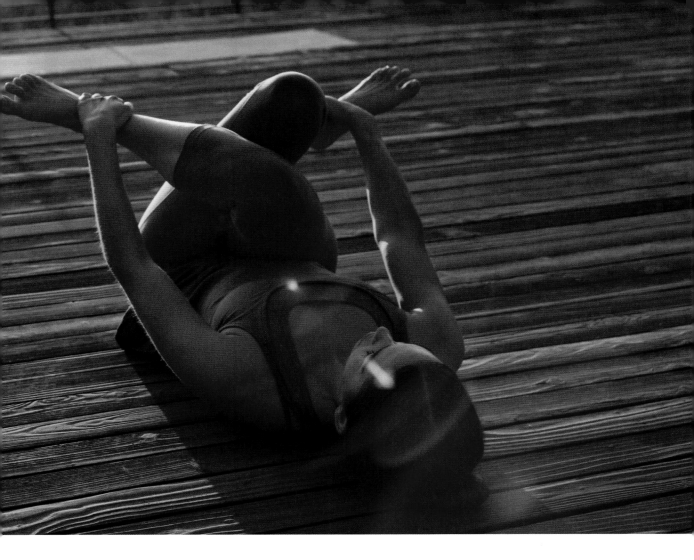

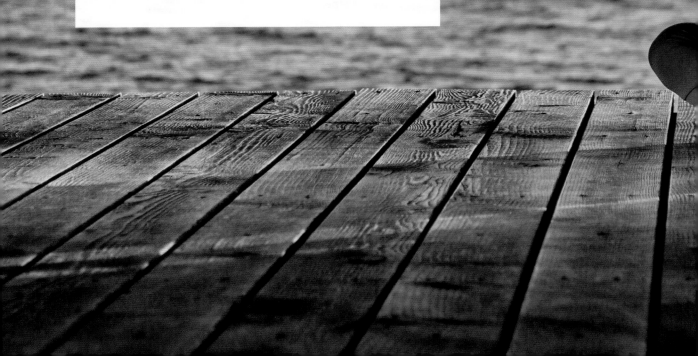

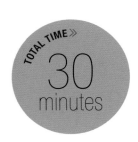
Neck & shoulder tension relief

This short sequence focuses on your neck and shoulders, and it can help eliminate kinks in your upper body. It might also support the healthy flow of energy through your heart and lung meridians as well as your throat chakra.

REQUIRED PROPS
• none

OPTIONAL PROPS
• 1 strap
• 1 block

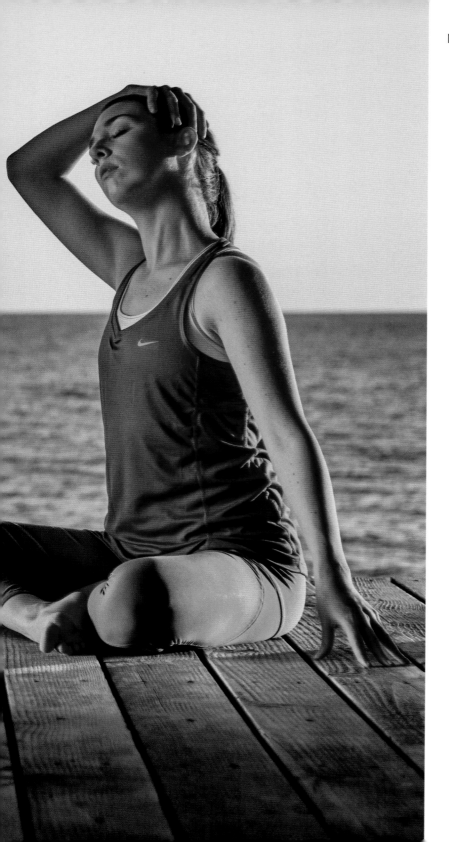

START

SEATED MEDITATION
page 24

hold for **3 mins**

NECK RELEASE
page 42

hold for **3 mins**
on each side

BOWTIE
page 108

hold for **3 mins**
on each side

ARCHER ARMS
page 64

hold for **3 mins**
on each side

LYING CHEST OPENER
page 56

hold for **3 mins**
on each side

CORPSE
page 144

hold for **3 mins**

FINISH

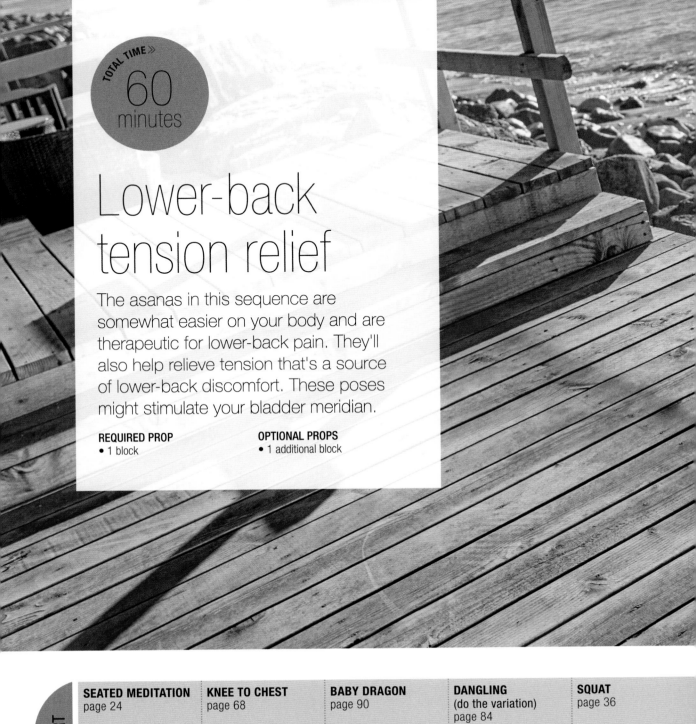

Lower-back tension relief

TOTAL TIME »
60 minutes

The asanas in this sequence are somewhat easier on your body and are therapeutic for lower-back pain. They'll also help relieve tension that's a source of lower-back discomfort. These poses might stimulate your bladder meridian.

REQUIRED PROP
• 1 block

OPTIONAL PROPS
• 1 additional block

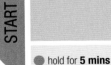

START

SEATED MEDITATION page 24	**KNEE TO CHEST** page 68	**BABY DRAGON** page 90	**DANGLING** (do the variation) page 84	**SQUAT** page 36
hold for **5 mins** »	hold for **5 mins** on each side »	hold for **5 mins** on each side »	hold for **5 mins** »	hold for **5 mins** »

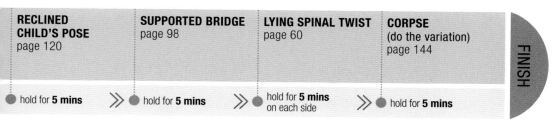

RECLINED CHILD'S POSE
page 120

SUPPORTED BRIDGE
page 98

LYING SPINAL TWIST
page 60

CORPSE
(do the variation)
page 144

FINISH

hold for **5 mins**   hold for **5 mins**   hold for **5 mins** on each side   hold for **5 mins**

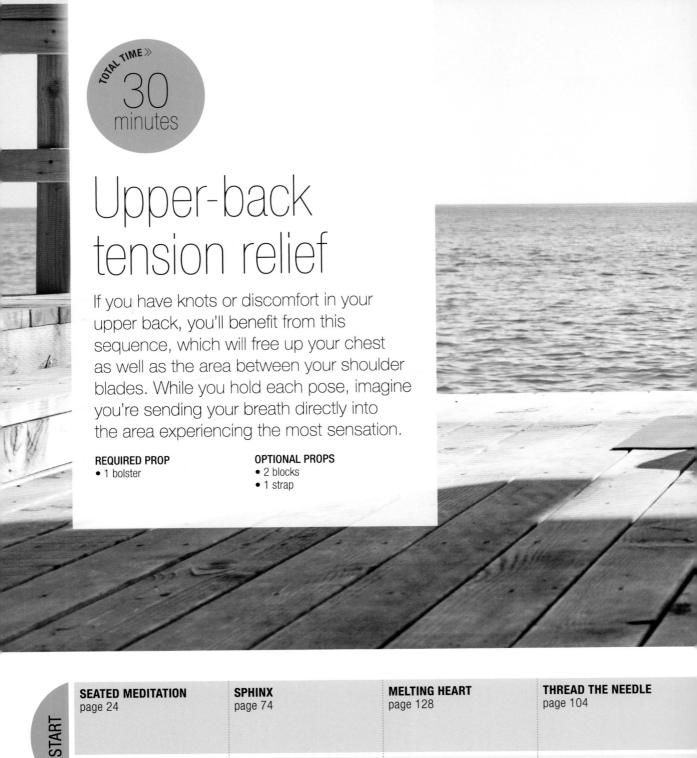

TOTAL TIME »

30 minutes

Upper-back tension relief

If you have knots or discomfort in your upper back, you'll benefit from this sequence, which will free up your chest as well as the area between your shoulder blades. While you hold each pose, imagine you're sending your breath directly into the area experiencing the most sensation.

REQUIRED PROP
- 1 bolster

OPTIONAL PROPS
- 2 blocks
- 1 strap

START

SEATED MEDITATION page 24	**SPHINX** page 74	**MELTING HEART** page 128	**THREAD THE NEEDLE** page 104
hold for **3 mins**	hold for **3 mins**	hold for **3 mins**	hold for **3 mins** on each side

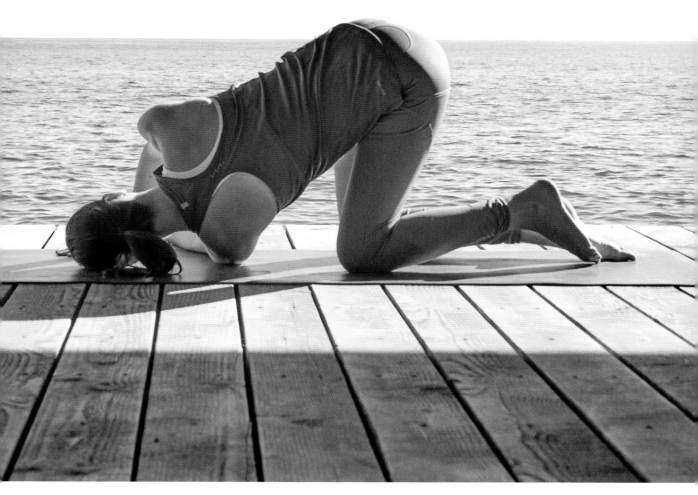

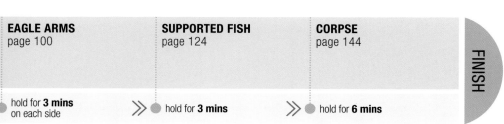

EAGLE ARMS
page 100

SUPPORTED FISH
page 124

CORPSE
page 144

FINISH

hold for **3 mins**
on each side

hold for **3 mins**

hold for **6 mins**

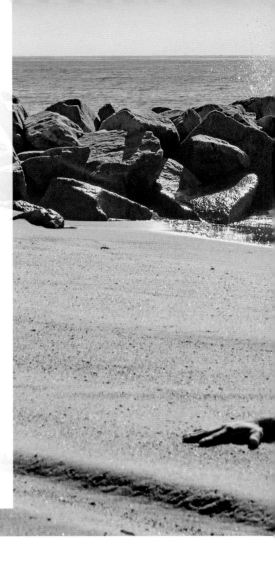

90 minutes

Advanced sequence

This sequence will take you through some more advanced asanas that will deeply stretch your spine, hips, and hamstrings. It's for more experienced yoga practitioners who already have good flexibility.

REQUIRED PROPS
• none

OPTIONAL PROPS
• 1 strap
• 2 blocks
• 1 bolster

START

SEATED MEDITATION page 24	**CATERPILLAR** page 48	**SHOELACE with ARCHER ARMS** pages 132 and 64	**STRADDLE** page 82
hold for **5 mins**	» hold for **10 mins**	» hold for **5 mins** on each side	» hold for **10 mins** »

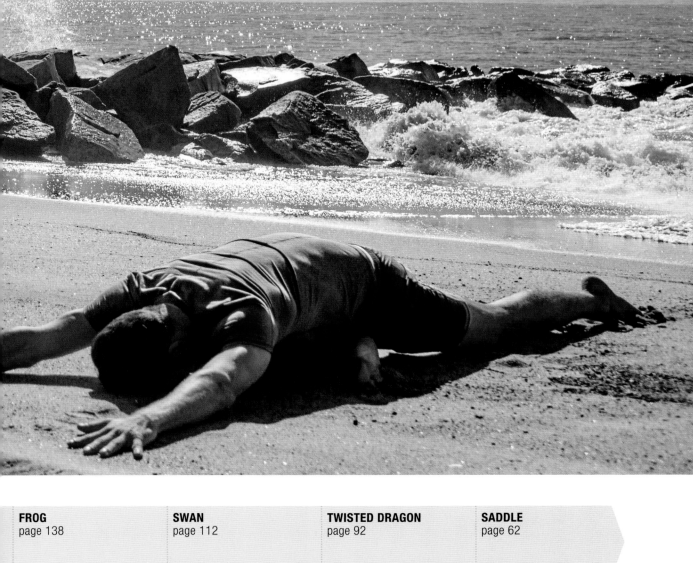

FROG page 138	**SWAN** page 112	**TWISTED DRAGON** page 92	**SADDLE** page 62
hold for **5 mins**	hold for **5 mins** on each side	hold for **5 mins** on each side	hold for **5 mins**

	SNAIL page 88	**LYING SPINAL TWIST** page 60	**CORPSE** page 144	FINISH
	hold for **5 mins**	hold for **5 mins** on each side	hold for **10 mins**	

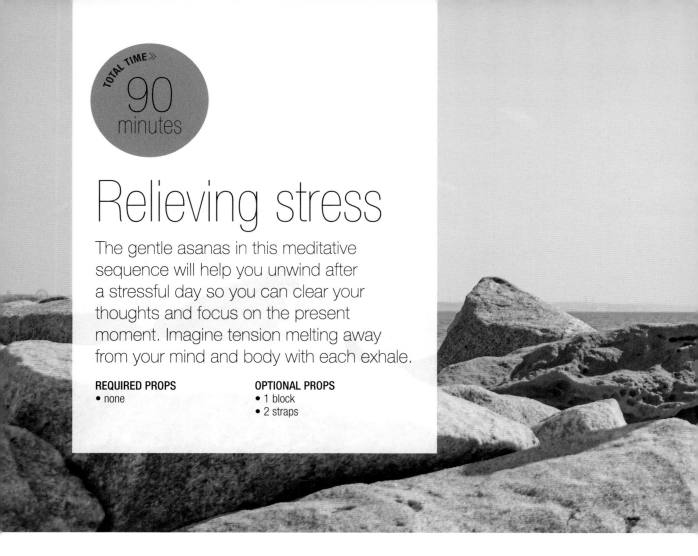

TOTAL TIME »

90 minutes

Relieving stress

The gentle asanas in this meditative sequence will help you unwind after a stressful day so you can clear your thoughts and focus on the present moment. Imagine tension melting away from your mind and body with each exhale.

REQUIRED PROPS
• none

OPTIONAL PROPS
• 1 block
• 2 straps

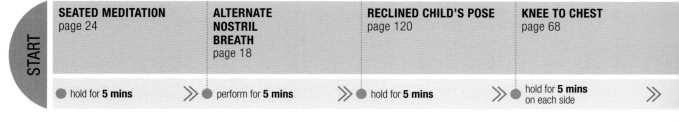

START

SEATED MEDITATION page 24	**ALTERNATE NOSTRIL BREATH** page 18	**RECLINED CHILD'S POSE** page 120	**KNEE TO CHEST** page 68
● hold for **5 mins**	● perform for **5 mins**	● hold for **5 mins**	● hold for **5 mins** on each side

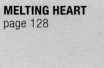

MELTING HEART page 128
● hold for **5 mins**

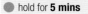

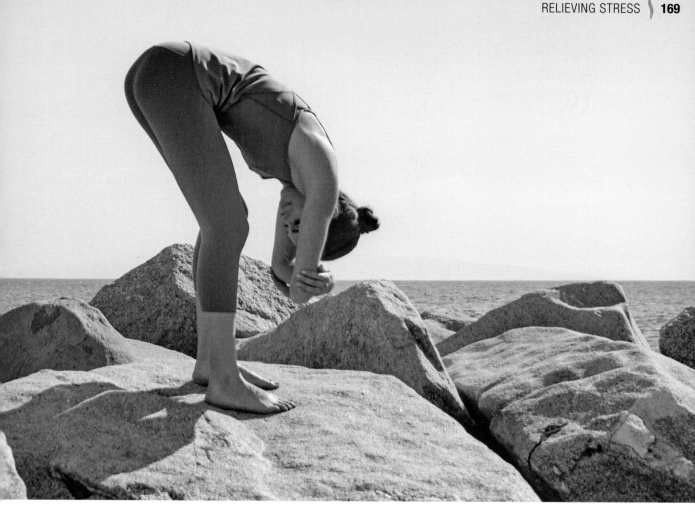

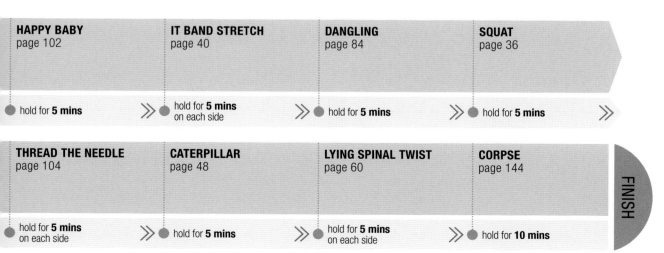

HAPPY BABY	IT BAND STRETCH	DANGLING	SQUAT
page 102	page 40	page 84	page 36
hold for **5 mins**	hold for **5 mins** on each side	hold for **5 mins**	hold for **5 mins**

THREAD THE NEEDLE	CATERPILLAR	LYING SPINAL TWIST	CORPSE	FINISH
page 104	page 48	page 60	page 144	
hold for **5 mins** on each side	hold for **5 mins**	hold for **5 mins** on each side	hold for **10 mins**	

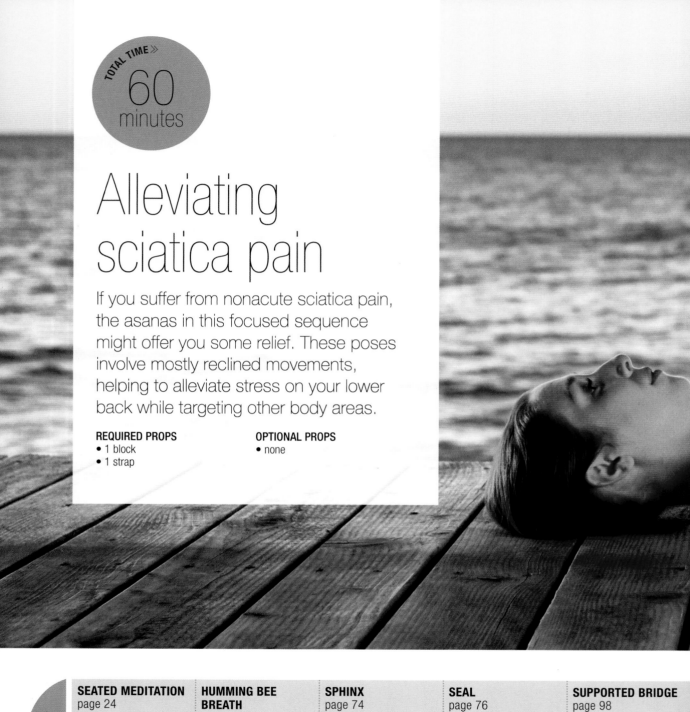

60 minutes

Alleviating sciatica pain

If you suffer from nonacute sciatica pain, the asanas in this focused sequence might offer you some relief. These poses involve mostly reclined movements, helping to alleviate stress on your lower back while targeting other body areas.

REQUIRED PROPS
- 1 block
- 1 strap

OPTIONAL PROPS
- none

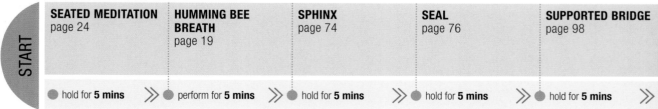

START

SEATED MEDITATION page 24	HUMMING BEE BREATH page 19	SPHINX page 74	SEAL page 76	SUPPORTED BRIDGE page 98
hold for **5 mins** »	perform for **5 mins** »	hold for **5 mins** »	hold for **5 mins** »	hold for **5 mins** »

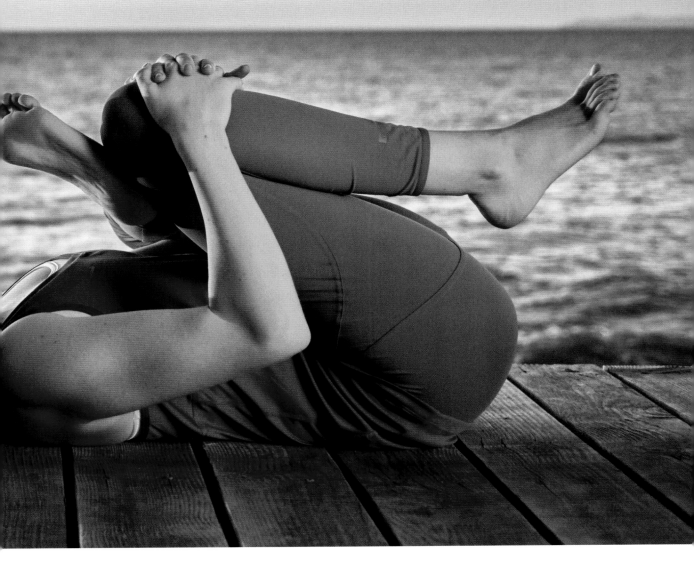

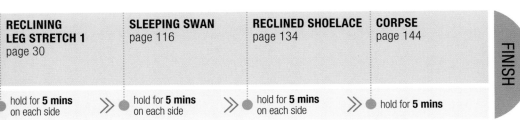

RECLINING LEG STRETCH 1 page 30	SLEEPING SWAN page 116	RECLINED SHOELACE page 134	CORPSE page 144	FINISH
hold for **5 mins** on each side	hold for **5 mins** on each side	hold for **5 mins** on each side	hold for **5 mins**	

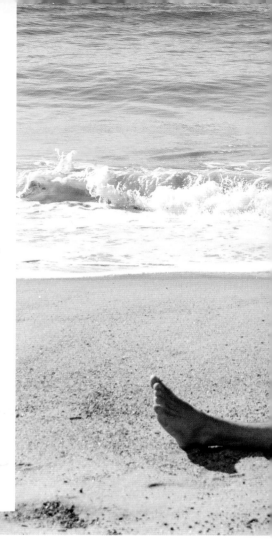

TOTAL TIME »

90 minutes

Increasing hamstring flexibility

This sequence focuses on the connective tissues around your hamstrings for increased flexibility in your lower body. These asanas will specifically target your legs, which can become overly stiff due to prolonged sitting.

REQUIRED PROPS
- 1 strap
- 1 block

OPTIONAL PROP
- 1 additional block

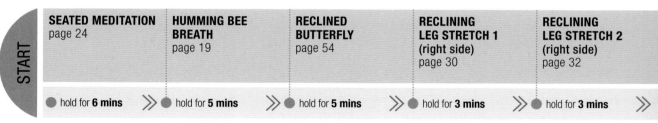

START

SEATED MEDITATION	**HUMMING BEE BREATH**	**RECLINED BUTTERFLY**	**RECLINING LEG STRETCH 1**	**RECLINING LEG STRETCH 2**
page 24	page 19	page 54	(right side) page 30	(right side) page 32
hold for **6 mins**	hold for **5 mins**	hold for **5 mins**	hold for **3 mins**	hold for **3 mins**

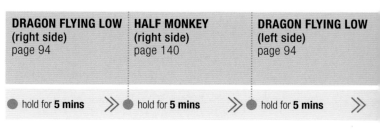

DRAGON FLYING LOW	**HALF MONKEY**	**DRAGON FLYING LOW**
(right side) page 94	(right side) page 140	(left side) page 94
hold for **5 mins**	hold for **5 mins**	hold for **5 mins**

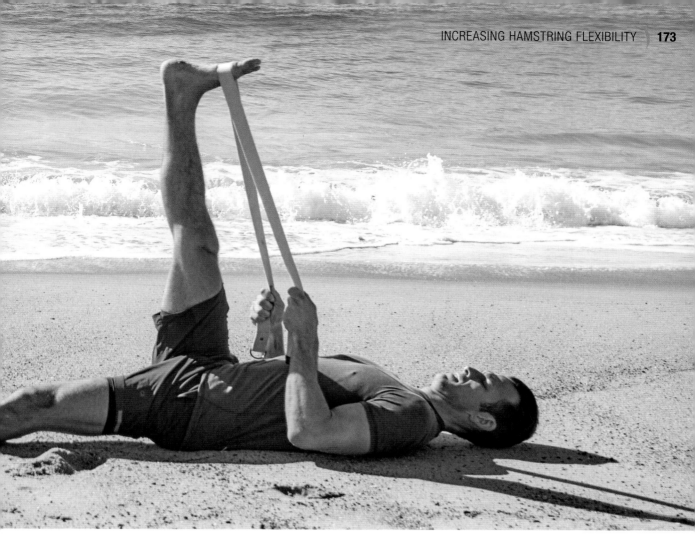

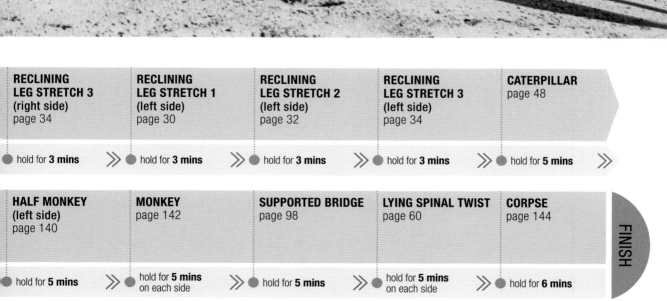

RECLINING LEG STRETCH 3
(right side)
page 34

hold for **3 mins** »

RECLINING LEG STRETCH 1
(left side)
page 30

hold for **3 mins** »

RECLINING LEG STRETCH 2
(left side)
page 32

hold for **3 mins** »

RECLINING LEG STRETCH 3
(left side)
page 34

hold for **3 mins** »

CATERPILLAR
page 48

hold for **5 mins** »

HALF MONKEY
(left side)
page 140

hold for **5 mins** »

MONKEY
page 142

hold for **5 mins**
on each side »

SUPPORTED BRIDGE
page 98

hold for **5 mins** »

LYING SPINAL TWIST
page 60

hold for **5 mins**
on each side »

CORPSE
page 144

hold for **6 mins**

FINISH

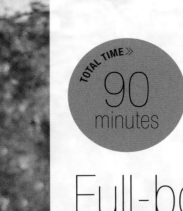

TOTAL TIME »

90 minutes

Full-body sequence

This sequence will remove stiffness from most joints, leaving you feeling refreshed and renewed. If you start to become distracted or disengaged, bring your awareness back to your breath and take your time going in and out of the poses.

REQUIRED PROPS
• none

OPTIONAL PROPS
• 2 blocks
• 1 strap

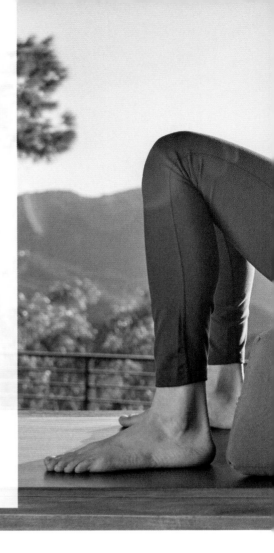

START

SEATED MEDITATION page 24	ALTERNATE NOSTRIL BREATH page 18	WRIST FLEXOR STRETCH page 70	WRIST EXTENSOR STRETCH page 72
hold for **4 mins** »	perform for **5 mins** »	hold for **3 mins** on each side »	hold for **3 mins** on each side »

HALF MONKEY page 140
hold for **5 mins** on each side »

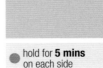

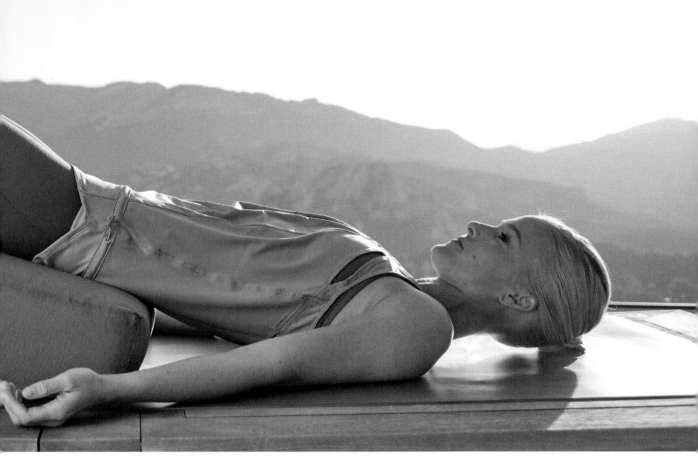

CHILD'S POSE page 118	BABY DRAGON page 90	LYING QUAD STRETCH page 58	SPHINX page 74
hold for **5 mins**	hold for **5 mins** on each side	hold for **5 mins** on each side	hold for **5 mins**

SADDLE page 62	LYING SPINAL TWIST page 60	LEGS UP THE WALL page 130	CORPSE page 144	FINISH
hold for **5 mins**	hold for **5 mins** on each side	hold for **10 mins**	hold for **4 mins**	

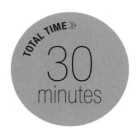

Side-body sequence

This sequence will help you open up the sides of your body—all the way from your neck down into your rib cage, hips, and outer leg—to begin to bring balance back to your entire body when you're short on time. You can work on your spinal flexibility and capacity for deep breathing by lengthening these tighter areas. This sequence might also stimulate your liver and gallbladder meridians.

REQUIRED PROPS
• none

OPTIONAL PROP
• 1 block

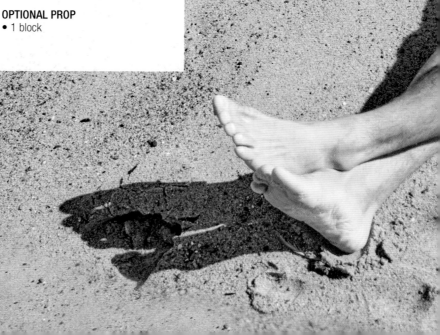

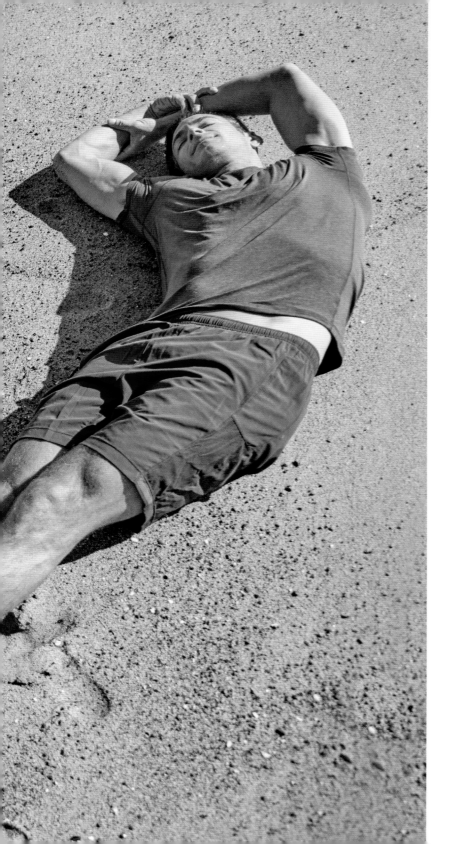

START

SEATED MEDITATION
page 24

hold for **3 mins**

NECK RELEASE
page 42

hold for **3 mins**
on each side

HALF BUTTERFLY
page 52

hold for **3 mins**
on each side

IT BAND STRETCH
page 40

hold for **3 mins**
on each side

BANANA
page 80

hold for **3 mins**
on each side

CORPSE
page 144

hold for **3 mins**

FINISH

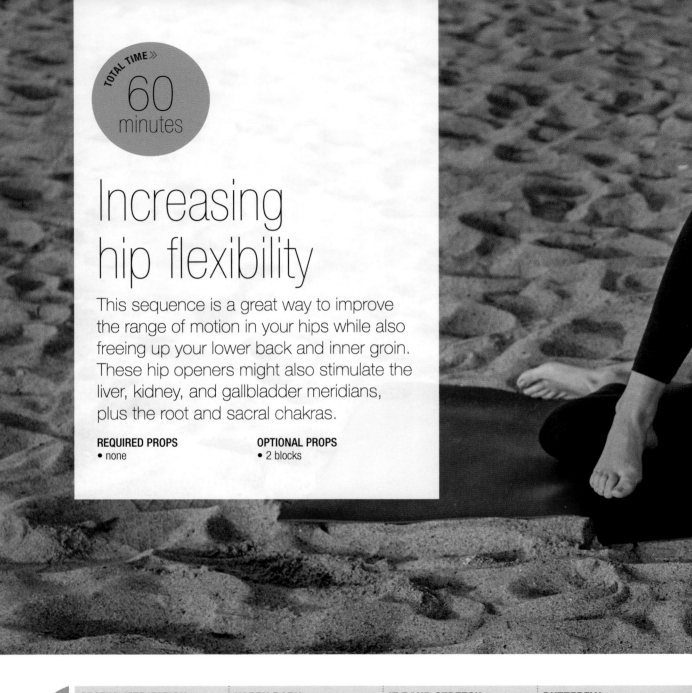

Increasing hip flexibility

This sequence is a great way to improve the range of motion in your hips while also freeing up your lower back and inner groin. These hip openers might also stimulate the liver, kidney, and gallbladder meridians, plus the root and sacral chakras.

TOTAL TIME »
60 minutes

REQUIRED PROPS
• none

OPTIONAL PROPS
• 2 blocks

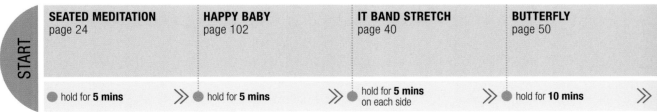

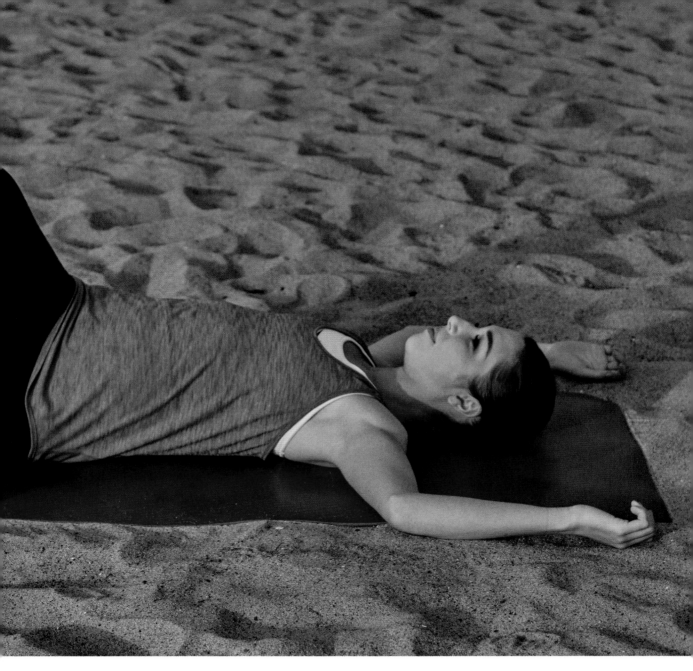

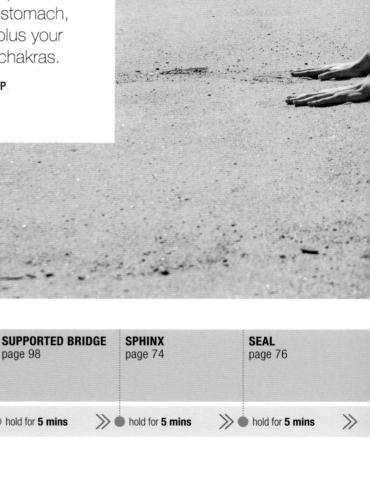

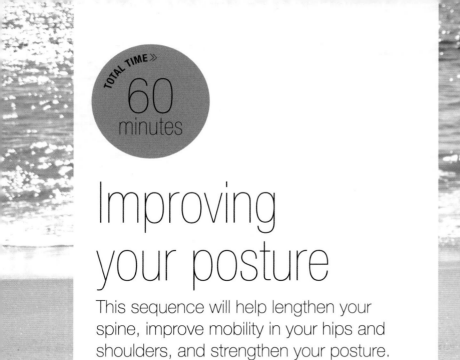

TOTAL TIME »

60
minutes

Improving
your posture

This sequence will help lengthen your spine, improve mobility in your hips and shoulders, and strengthen your posture. The energetic focus is on your stomach, kidney, and spleen meridians, plus your sacral, solar plexus, and heart chakras.

REQUIRED PROP
• 1 block

OPTIONAL PROP
• 1 block

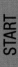

START

SEATED MEDITATION page 24	KNEE TO CHEST page 68	SUPPORTED BRIDGE page 98	SPHINX page 74	SEAL page 76
hold for **5 mins**	hold for **5 mins** on each side	hold for **5 mins**	hold for **5 mins**	hold for **5 mins**

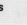

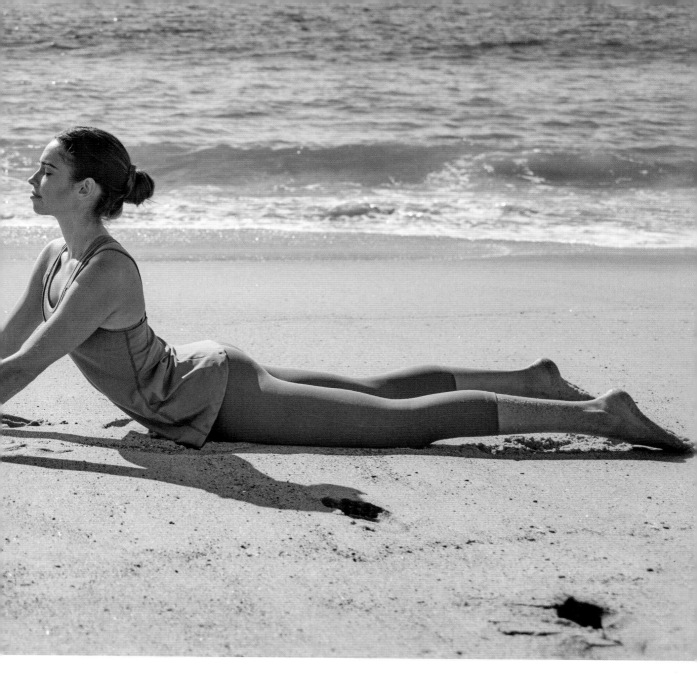

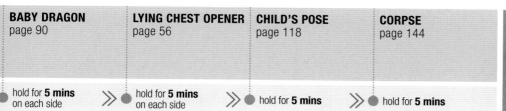

BABY DRAGON page 90	**LYING CHEST OPENER** page 56	**CHILD'S POSE** page 118	**CORPSE** page 144	FINISH
hold for **5 mins** on each side	hold for **5 mins** on each side	hold for **5 mins**	hold for **5 mins**	

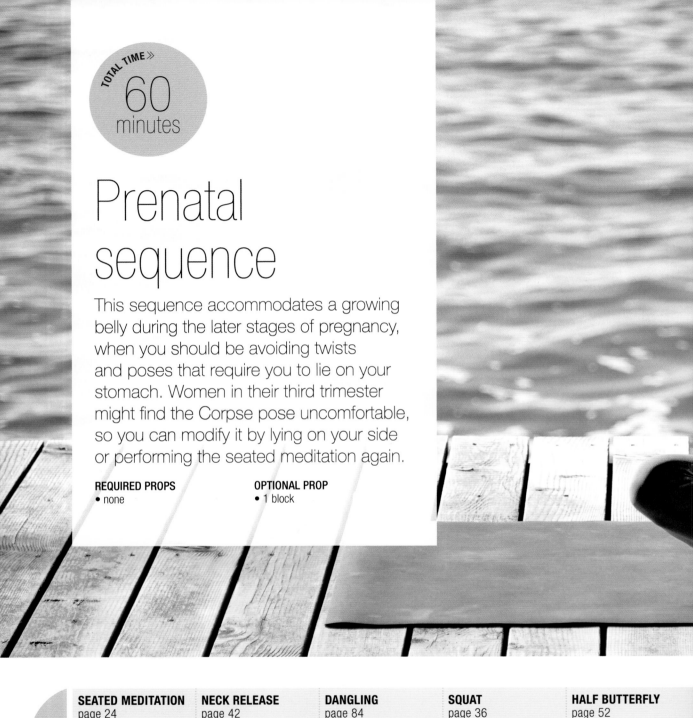

Prenatal sequence

This sequence accommodates a growing belly during the later stages of pregnancy, when you should be avoiding twists and poses that require you to lie on your stomach. Women in their third trimester might find the Corpse pose uncomfortable, so you can modify it by lying on your side or performing the seated meditation again.

REQUIRED PROPS
• none

OPTIONAL PROP
• 1 block

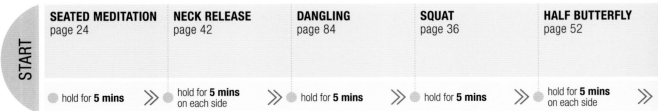

START

SEATED MEDITATION page 24	**NECK RELEASE** page 42	**DANGLING** page 84	**SQUAT** page 36	**HALF BUTTERFLY** page 52
hold for **5 mins** »	hold for **5 mins** on each side »	hold for **5 mins** »	hold for **5 mins** »	hold for **5 mins** on each side »

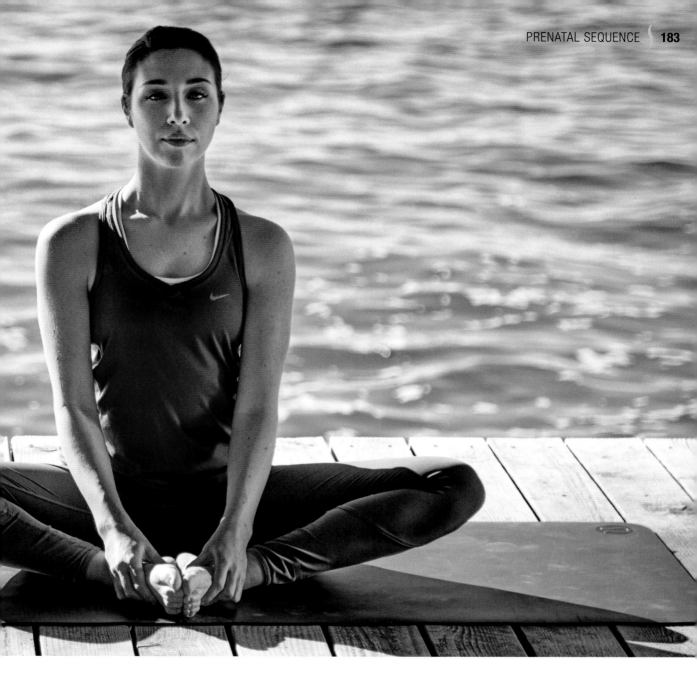

BUTTERFLY page 50	ANKLE STRETCH page 44	SEAL page 76	CHILD'S POSE (do the variation) page 118	CORPSE (on your side) page 144 or SEATED MEDITATION page 24	FINISH
hold for **5 mins**	hold for **3 mins** on each side	hold for **3 mins**	hold for **5 mins**	hold for **6 mins**	

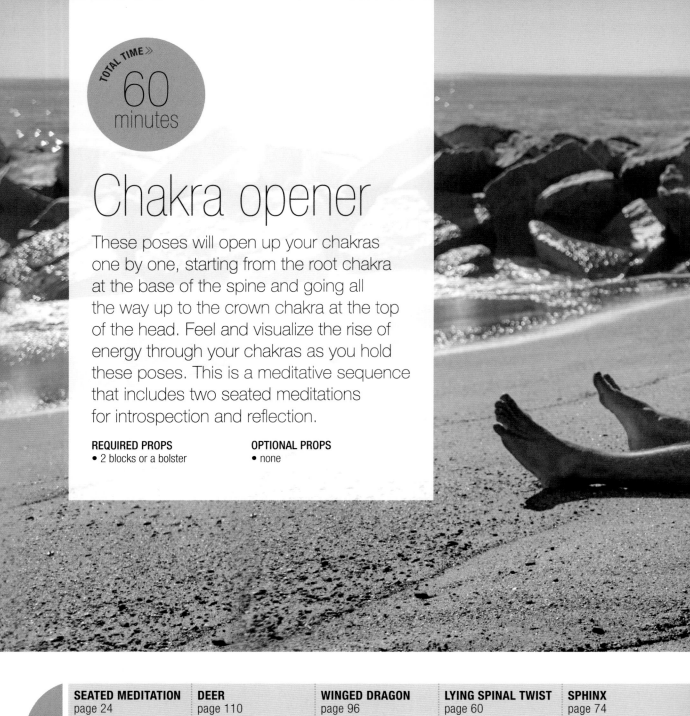

60 minutes

Chakra opener

These poses will open up your chakras one by one, starting from the root chakra at the base of the spine and going all the way up to the crown chakra at the top of the head. Feel and visualize the rise of energy through your chakras as you hold these poses. This is a meditative sequence that includes two seated meditations for introspection and reflection.

REQUIRED PROPS
• 2 blocks or a bolster

OPTIONAL PROPS
• none

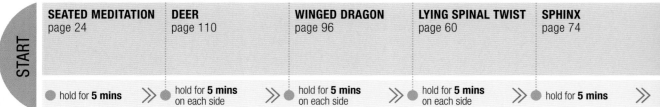

START

SEATED MEDITATION page 24	**DEER** page 110	**WINGED DRAGON** page 96	**LYING SPINAL TWIST** page 60	**SPHINX** page 74
hold for **5 mins**	hold for **5 mins** on each side	hold for **5 mins** on each side	hold for **5 mins** on each side	hold for **5 mins**

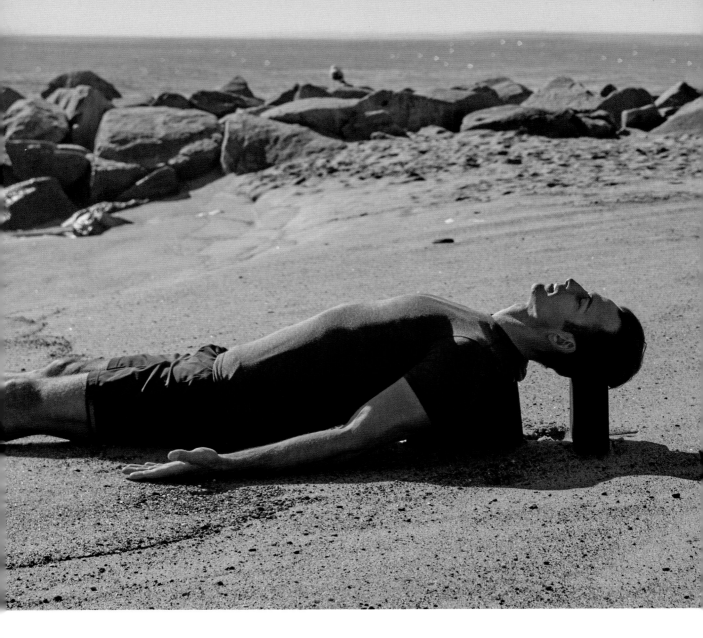

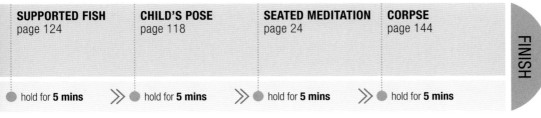

SUPPORTED FISH page 124	**CHILD'S POSE** page 118	**SEATED MEDITATION** page 24	**CORPSE** page 144	FINISH
hold for **5 mins**	hold for **5 mins**	hold for **5 mins**	hold for **5 mins**	

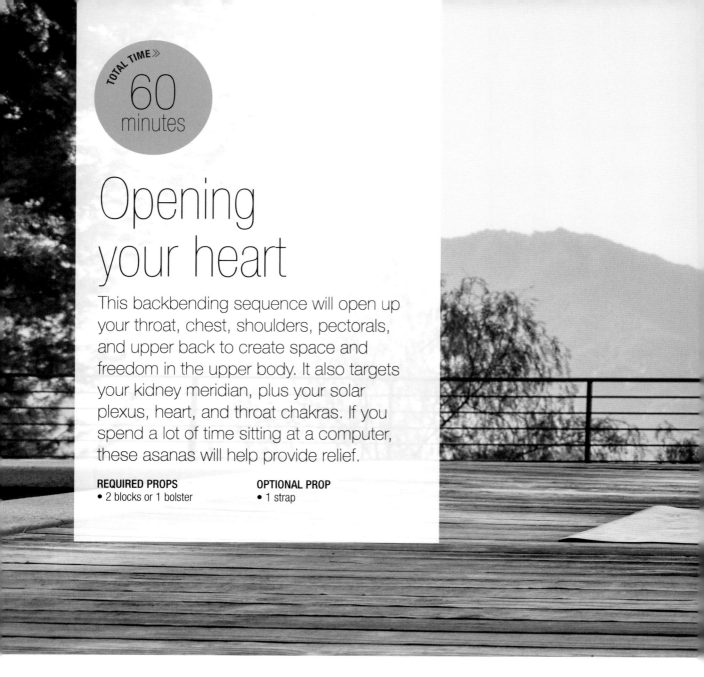

TOTAL TIME »

60
minutes

Opening
your heart

This backbending sequence will open up your throat, chest, shoulders, pectorals, and upper back to create space and freedom in the upper body. It also targets your kidney meridian, plus your solar plexus, heart, and throat chakras. If you spend a lot of time sitting at a computer, these asanas will help provide relief.

REQUIRED PROPS
• 2 blocks or 1 bolster

OPTIONAL PROP
• 1 strap

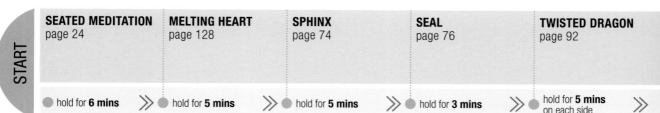

START

SEATED MEDITATION page 24	MELTING HEART page 128	SPHINX page 74	SEAL page 76	TWISTED DRAGON page 92
hold for **6 mins**	hold for **5 mins**	hold for **5 mins**	hold for **3 mins**	hold for **5 mins** on each side

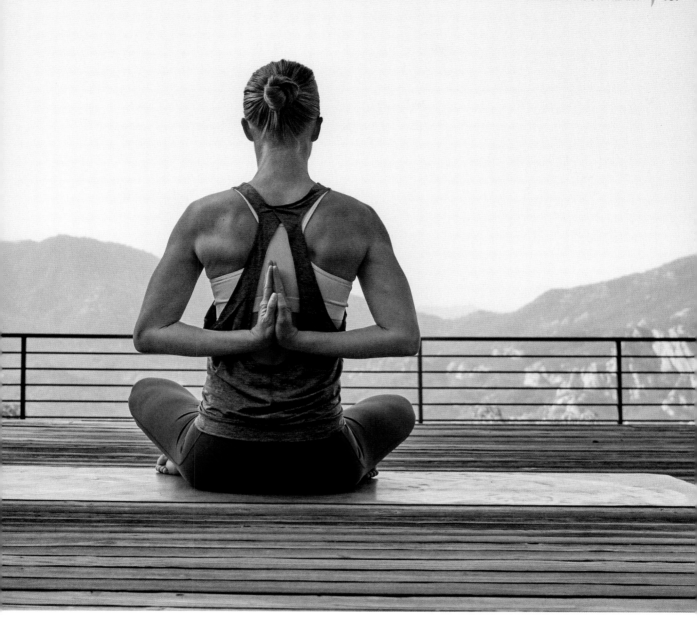

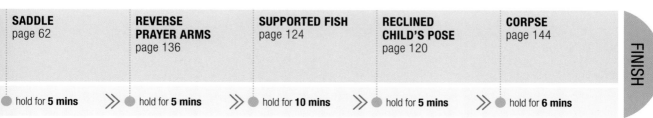

SADDLE
page 62

**REVERSE
PRAYER ARMS**
page 136

SUPPORTED FISH
page 124

**RECLINED
CHILD'S POSE**
page 120

CORPSE
page 144

FINISH

hold for **5 mins**   hold for **5 mins**   hold for **10 mins**   hold for **5 mins**   hold for **6 mins**

Index

About the author

Kassandra Reinhardt is an Ottawa-based yoga teacher and a leading online yin yoga instructor. Her "Yoga with Kassandra" YouTube channel has served as the gateway for thousands of people across the globe to discover the life-changing benefits of a consistent yin yoga practice. Kassandra first practiced yin yoga in 2008 as a way to become more flexible and to better learn to manage stress and anxiety. The effects were so profound that she knew she wanted to become a teacher and share the same tools with others. She's passionate about sharing the gifts of yin yoga with practitioners from all around the world. Practice with her today by visiting her website at www.yogawithkassandra.com.

Acknowledgments

Thanks to everyone at DK Books for making my dream of becoming a published author a reality. Working with you has been an experience that I'll never forget. I'd especially like to thank Christopher Stolle and Brook Farling for their dedication and support throughout this process. Thank you for being open to my ideas and giving me a voice.

A big thank you to our photoshoot art director Nigel Wright and photographer Christopher Malcolm for making this book the stunning work of art that it is. Along with our fantastic models—Kelly Collins, Ryan Young, Brittany Martinez, and Q Brandon—you made the photo shoot feel like an exciting collaboration with friends, no matter how long the hours were. There was never a dull moment on set, and I appreciate your dedication and attention to detail.

A heartfelt thanks goes to my family and friends, who never cease to encourage me and are always there to lend an ear when I need it. You continuously inspire me to push myself and remind me that I can do anything I set my mind to.

Finally, I want to acknowledge my partner-in-crime, Anthony, without whom none of this would've been possible. Thank you for always being at my side, cheering me on, and believing in me even when I don't believe in myself. For standing by my side during the ups and downs and loving me through it all, this is for you.

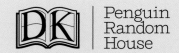

Publisher: Mike Sanders
Associate Publisher: Billy Fields
Senior Editor: Brook Farling
Editor: Christopher Stolle
Cover Designer: Nicola Powling
Book Designer: Hannah Moore
Photoshoot Art Director: Nigel Wright
Photographer: Christopher Malcolm
Prepress Technician: Brian Massey
Proofreader: Laura Caddell
Indexer: Heather McNeill

First American Edition 2017
Published in the United States by
DK Publishing, 6081 E. 82nd Street, Indianapolis, Indiana 46250

ISBN: 978-1-46546-273-2
Library of Congress Catalog Card Number: 2017939981